Anaesthesia at a Glance

Julian Stone

Consultant Anaesthetist
Great Western Hospital NHS Foundation Trust
Swindon, UK;
Senior Clinical Lecturer
University of Bristol
Bristol, UK

William Fawcett

...undation Trust;

Post~.duate Medic~. ~chool
University of Surrey
Guildford, UK

WILEY Blackwell

This edition first published 2013 © 2013 by Julian Stone and William Fawcett.

Registered office: John Wiley & Sons, Ltd, The Atrium, Southern Gate, Chichester, West Sussex, PO19 8SQ, UK

Editorial offices: 9600 Garsington Road, Oxford, OX4 2DQ, UK

The Atrium, Southern Gate, Chichester, West Sussex, PO19 8SQ, UK

111 River Street, Hoboken, NJ 07030-5774, USA

For details of our global editorial offices, for customer services and for information about how to apply for permission to reuse the copyright material in this book please see our website at www.wiley.com/wiley-blackwell

Library of Congress Cataloging-in-Publication Data
Stone, Julian, author.
Anaesthesia at a glance / Julian Stone, William Fawcett.
p. ; cm. – (At a glance)
Includes bibliographical references and index.
ISBN 978-1-4051-8756-5 (pbk. : alk. paper) – ISBN 978-1-118-76533-3 (ePub) – ISBN 978-1-118-76532-6 – ISBN 978-1-118-76531-9 – ISBN 978-1-118-76530-2 (Mobi) – ISBN 978-1-118-76529-6
I. Fawcett, William, 1962– author. II. Title. III. Series: At a glance series (Oxford, England)
[DNLM: 1. Anesthesia–methods. 2. Anesthesiology–instrumentation. 3. Anesthetics. WO 200]
RD81
617.9′6–dc23

2013018954

A catalogue record for this book is available from the British Library.

Wiley also publishes its books in a variety of electronic formats. Some content that appears in print may not be available in electronic books.

Cover image: © iStockphoto/Beerkoff
Cover design by Meaden Creative

Set in 9 on 11.5 pt Times by Toppan Best-set Premedia Limited
Printed and bound in Malaysia by Vivar Printing Sdn Bhd

1 2013

Contents

Preface

Anaesthesia is often intimidating for students. Within the relatively short time allocated to this disciplines on most undergraduate curricula, there seems to be a bewildering array of unfamiliar drugs, equipment and practical procedures. Yet at the very heart of anaesthesia is the modern concept of perioperative medicine. The fundamentals of anaesthesia, such as assessment and management of the airway, respiration, circulation and analgesia, are applicable to all hospital staff involved in the care of the surgical patient.

Both authors are practising clinical anaesthetists and also actively involved in undergraduate teaching. Moreover, as anaesthetists are the largest single group of doctors within hospital medicine it seems appropriate that a contemporary undergraduate textbook is available as an introduction to the specialty.

The aim of the authors has been to cover the practice of anaesthesia to a level appropriate for a medical student who is about to embark on the Foundation Programme. Certain specialized subjects that are traditionally taught, such as physics, have therefore been omitted.

Each chapter has a self assessment section of both multiple choice questions and case studies. The answers are not exhaustive, but should encourage further reading on the subject.

Whilst this book is aimed primarily at undergraduate medical students, it may also prove of value to Foundation Doctors looking after patients in the perioperative period, doctors embarking on a career in anaesthesia and theatre staff such as Operating Department Practitioners

The authors would like to thank Laura Murphy, Helen Harvey, Elizabeth Norton, Simon Jones, Ruth Swan, Kevin Fung and Brenda Sibbald. They acknowledge and dedicate this book to those who have given encouragement and support throughout. JS would like to thank Edwina, Freddie, Hugo and Lucinda. WF would like to thank Victoria, George, Alice and Joseph.

Julian Stone
William Fawcett

How to use your textbook

Features contained within your textbook

Each topic is presented in a double-page spread with clear, easy-to-follow diagrams supported by succinct explanatory text.

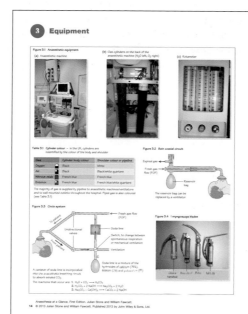

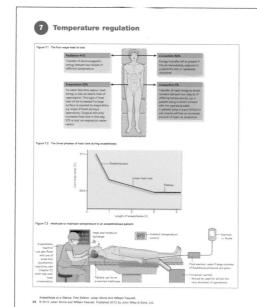

The anytime, anywhere textbook

Wiley E-Text

Your book is also available to purchase as a **Wiley E-Text: Powered by VitalSource** version – a digital, interactive version of this book which you own as soon as you download it.

Your **Wiley E-Text** allows you to:

Search: Save time by finding terms and topics instantly in your book, your notes, even your whole library (once you've downloaded more textbooks)

Note and Highlight: Colour code, highlight and make digital notes right in the text so you can find them quickly and easily

Organize: Keep books, notes and class materials organized in folders inside the application

Share: Exchange notes and highlights with friends, classmates and study groups

Upgrade: Your textbook can be transferred when you need to change or upgrade computers

Link: Link directly from the page of your interactive textbook to all of the material contained on the companion website

The **Wiley E-Text** version will also allow you to copy and paste any photograph or illustration into assignments, presentations and your own notes.

To access your Wiley E-Text

- Visit **www.vitalsource.com/software/bookshelf/downloads** to download the Bookshelf application to your computer, laptop or mobile device.
- Open the Bookshelf application on your computer and register for an account.
- Follow the registration process.

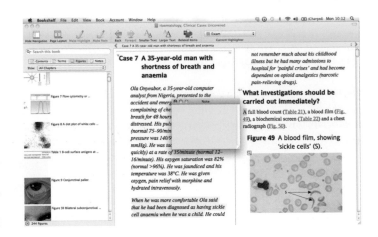

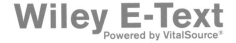

The VitalSource Bookshelf can now be used to view your Wiley E-Text **on iOS, Android and Kindle Fire!**

- For iOS: Visit the app store to download the VitalSource Bookshelf: https://itunes.apple.com/gb/app/vitalsource-bookshelf/id389359495?mt=8
- For Android: Visit the Google Play Market to download the VitalSource Bookshelf: http://support.vitalsource.com/kb/android/getting-started
- For Kindle Fire, Kindle Fire 2 or Kindle Fire HD: Simply install the VitalSource Bookshelf onto your Fire (see how at http://support.vitalsource.com/kb/Kindle-Fire/app-installation-guide). You can now sign in with the email address and password you used when you created your VitalSource Bookshelf Account.

  Full E-Text support for mobile devices is available at: http://support.vitalsource.com

CourseSmart

CourseSmart gives you instant access (via computer or mobile device) to this Wiley-Blackwell e-book and its extra electronic functionality, at 40% off the recommended retail print price. See all the benefits at: **www.coursesmart.com/students**

Instructors . . . receive your own digital desk copies!

CourseSmart also offers instructors an immediate, efficient, and environmentally-friendly way to review this book for your course.

For more information visit www.coursesmart.com/instructors.

With CourseSmart, you can create lecture notes quickly with copy and paste, and share pages and notes with your students. Access your **CourseSmart** digital book from your computer or mobile device instantly for evaluation, class preparation, and as a teaching tool in the classroom.

Simply sign in at **http://instructors.coursesmart.com/bookshelf** to download your Bookshelf and get started. To request your desk copy, hit 'Request Online Copy' on your search results or book product page.

We hope you enjoy using your new book. Good luck with your studies!

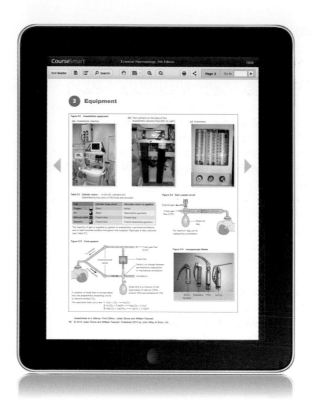

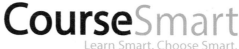

About the companion website

This book is accompanied by a companion website:

 www.ataglanceseries.com/anaesthesia

The website includes:
• Interactive MCQs
• Interactive case studies

Abbreviations

ABC	airway, breathing and circulation
AICD	automated implantable cardioverter-defibrillator
APL	adjustable pressure-limiting valve
ASA	American Society of Anesthesiologists
AT	anaerobic threshold
ATLS	advanced trauma life support
AVPU	alert, verbal, pain, unresponsive
BCIS	bone cement implantation syndrome
BMI	body mass index
BP	blood pressure
<C>ABC	catastrophic haemorrhage, airway, breathing and circulation
CABG	coronary artery bypass graft
CBT	cognitive behavioural therapy
CC	closing capacity
CGO	common gas outlet
CMRO$_2$	cerebral metabolic requirement for oxygen
CNS	central nervous system
CO	cardiac output
COPA	cuffed oropharyngeal airway
COPD	chronic obstructive pulmonary disease
CPAP	continuous positive airway pressure
CPB	cardiopulmonary bypass
CPET	cardiopulmonary exercise testing
CRPS	complex regional pain syndrome
CSE	combined spinal epidural
CT	computed tomography
CVA	cerebrovascular accident
CVCI	can't ventilate can't intubate
CVP	central venous pressure
CVS	cardiovascular system
DHCA	deep hypothermic circulatory arrest
DKA	diabetic ketoacidosis
DLT	double-lumen tube
DRG	dorsal root ganglion
DVT	deep venous thrombosis
ECG	electrocardiogram
ECT	electroconvulsive therapy
EMLA	eutectic mixture of local anaesthetics
ESR	erythrocyte sedimentation rate
ETCO$_2$	end tidal CO$_2$
ETT	endotracheal tube
EVAR	endovascular aneurysm repair
EWS	early warning scores
FES	fat embolism syndrome
FGF	fresh gas flow
FMS	fibromyalgia syndrome
FRC	functional residual capacity
FRCA	Fellowship of the Royal College of Anaesthetists
GA	general anaesthetic
GABA	γ-aminobutyric acid
GIK	glucose, insulin and potassium
HDU	high dependency unit
HR	heart rate
IBW	ideal body weight
ICM	intensive care medicine
ICU	intensive care unit
ILMA	intubating laryngeal mask airway
INR	international normalized ratio
IO	intraosseous
IOP	intraocular pressure
IPPV	intermittent positive pressure ventilation
IVC	inferior vena cava
IVRA	intravenous regional anaesthesia
LA	local anaesthetic
LiDCO	A device for measuring cardiac output continuously from an arterial line using lithium dilution
LMA	laryngeal mask airway
LV	left ventricle
LVEDP	left ventricular end diastolic pressure
LVEDV	left ventricular end diastolic volume
MAC	minimum alveolar concentration
MEOWS	modified early obstetric warning scores
MERT	medical emergency response team
MEWS	modified early warning scores
MFS	myofascial syndrome
MH	malignant hyperthermia
MI	myocardial ischaemia
MRI	magnet resonance imaging
NCA	nurse-controlled analgesia
NIDDM	non-insulin-dependent diabetes mellitus
NIST	non-interchangeable screw thread
NMBD	neuromuscular blocking drug
NMDA	N-methyl-D-aspartate
NSAID	non-steroid anti-inflammatory drug
OLA	one-lung anaesthesia
OSA	obstructive sleep apnoea
PCA	patient-controlled analgesia
PCI	percutaneous coronary intervention
POCD	postoperative cognitive dysfunction
PONV	postoperative nausea and vomiting
RAE	Ring–Adair–Elwyn tube
RS	respiratory system
RVEDP	right ventricular end diastolic pressure
SSRI	selective serotonin reuptake inhibitor
SVC	superior vena cava
SVR	systemic vascular resistance
TENS	transcutaneous electrical nerve stimulation
TIA	transient ischaemic attack
TIVA	total intravenous anaesthesia
U&E	urea and electrolytes
URTI	upper respiratory tract infection
UTI	urinary tract infection
VIE	vacuum insulated evaporator
VQ	ventilation–perfusion

History of anaesthesia

Figure 1.1 Timeline

1772	– Nitrous oxide (N_2O) described and synthesized by Joseph Priestly
1798	– Humphrey Davy used N_2O experimentally
1844	– Horace Wells performed the first public demonstration of N_2O in December 1844
1863	– N_2O entered general dental practice
1846	– William Morton used ether at Massachusetts General Hospital, Boston in October 1846. Dr Oliver Holmes, who was present, described the state induced by ether as 'anaesthesia'
1846	– Ether used in Dumfries and London
1847	– James Simpson introduced chloroform
1853	– John Snow administered chloroform to Queen Victoria during the birth of Prince Leopold – Joseph Clover developed anaesthesia as a medical specialty – Chloroform was replaced due to its toxicity
1884	– Carl Koller described the use of topical cocaine
1884	– William Halstead and Richard Hall injected local anaesthetic into tissue and nerves
1885	– Leonard Corning described spinal anaesthesia in dogs
1885	– Walter Essex Wyntner and Heinrich Quincke independently described dural puncture
1899	– Gustav Bier performed spinal anaesthesia
1902	– Henry Cushing described regional anaesthesia
1907	– Continuous spinal anaesthesia described
1921	– Fidel Pagés Miravé (a Spanish surgeon) described epidural anaesthesia
1920s	– Intubation of the larynx developed
1935	– Ralph Waters and John Lundy independently used thiopentone as an intravenous induction agent
1942	– Neuromuscular blocking drugs first used in surgical operations by Harold Griffith and Enid Johnson
1949	– Martinez Curbelo (Cuba) administered the first continuous epidural anaesthetic (continuous spinal anaesthesia had originally been described in 1907)
1950s	– Halothane introduced: its smooth induction, pleasant smell and potency proved advantageous. It needed new vaporizer technology, allowing more accurate dose administration
1977	– Propofol introduced as an induction agent, allowing smooth induction and rapid recovery with minimal hangover effect
1980s	– Laryngeal Mask Airway (LMA) introduced by British anaesthetist Archie Brain, resulting in a marked reduction in the number of patients being intubated during anaesthesia. It has since become a key aid in patients who are difficult to intubate as well as rescue techniques when failure to intubate and/or ventilate a patient occurs
1948	– The Faculty of Anaesthetists of the Royal College of Surgeons founded
1988	– The College of Anaesthetists founded as part of the Royal College of Surgeons
1992	– Royal Charter granted to the Royal College of Anaesthetists

Anaesthesia at a Glance, First Edition. Julian Stone and William Fawcett.

Before the introduction of anaesthesia, it would not have been possible to carry out the majority of modern operations. Development of the triad of hypnosis, analgesia and muscle relaxation has enabled surgery to be performed that would otherwise be inconceivable.

Early attempts at pain reduction included the use of opium (described in Homer's Odyssey 700 BC), alcohol and coca leaves (these were chewed by Inca shamans and their saliva used for its local anaesthetic effect).

Attempts at relieving childbirth pain could (and did) result in accusations of witchcraft.

If surgery had to be performed, it usually involved restraint, administration of alcohol and the procedure being performed as quickly as possible (amputations often took a matter of seconds).

Nitrous oxide (N_2O) was described and first synthesized by Joseph Priestly in 1772. It was used experimentally by Humphry Davy, who also introduced its use to London intellectuals at the time, such as the poet Samuel Taylor Coleridge, engineer James Watt and potter Josiah Wedgewood. Priestly also discovered oxygen, describing it as 'dephlogisticated air'.

First documented anaesthetic

The first *documented* use of N_2O was in North America, by Horace Wells (a dentist) in Hartford, Connecticut in December 1844, for a dental extraction in front of a medical audience. The patient cried out during the procedure (although later denied feeling any pain) and Wells was discredited, never to fully recover and eventually committing suicide.

N_2O subsequently entered general dental practice in 1863.

Ether and chloroform

In October 1846, William Morton (also a dentist) used ether at the Massachusetts General Hospital, Boston during an operation on a neck tumour, performed by surgeon John Warren. Dr Oliver Holmes, who was present, described the state induced by ether as 'anaesthesia'.

On 19th December 1846, ether was used in Dumfries (during a limb amputation of a patient who had been run over by a cart) and in London (for a tooth extraction).

James Simpson (Professor of Obstetrics in Edinburgh) introduced chloroform in November 1847, having discovered its effectiveness at a dinner party held at his house on 4th November that year.

John Snow administered chloroform to Queen Victoria during the birth of Prince Leopold *(chloroform a la reine)*. Her positive endorsement of pain relief during labour removed religious objections to the practice at that time. (Snow is also famous for his epidemiological work, which identified the Broad Street water pump as the source of a cholera epidemic in London in 1854, confirming it as a water-borne disease.)

Chloroform was later replaced due to its toxicity and potential to cause fatal cardiac dysrhythmias.

Anaesthesia as a medical specialty

The development of anaesthesia as a specialty has been attributed to Joseph Clover. He advocated examining the patient before giving an anaesthetic as well as palpating a pulse throughout the duration of anaesthesia. He described cricothrotomy as a means of treating airway obstruction during 'chloroform asphyxia'.

The development and use of local anaesthetics

Carl Koller (an ophthalmologist from Vienna) described the use of topical cocaine for analgesia of the eye in 1884, having been given a sample by his friend Sigmund Freud (the founder of modern-day psychoanalysis) who worked in the same hospital.

In 1884, William Halstead and Richard Hall, in New York, injected local anaesthetic into tissue and nerves to produce analgesia for surgery. The following year, also in New York, Leonard Corning, a neurologist, described cocaine spinal anaesthesia in dogs; he had inadvertently performed an epidural block. Six months later, Walter Essex Wyntner in the UK and Heinrich Quincke in Germany independently described dural puncture (this was used for the treatment of hydrocephalus secondary to tubercular meningitis).

In 1899, Gustav Bier performed spinal anaesthesia on six patients as well as on his assistant – who also performed the same procedure on Bier. They tested the efficacy of the anaesthetic on each other with lit cigars and hammers. Both reported significant post dural puncture headache, which at the time they attributed to too much alcohol consumed in celebration of their achievement. He also described intravenous regional anaesthesia (IVRA), in which local anaesthetic is injected intravenously (usually prilocaine) in a limb vein, with proximal spread prevented by a tourniquet – the Bier's block.

In 1902, Henry Cushing described regional anaesthesia (blocking large nerve plexi under direct vision in patients receiving a general anaesthetic).

The Spanish surgeon Fidel Pagés Miravé described epidural anaesthesia for surgery in 1921.

Typical career path in anaesthesia

- Medical School: 5–6 years;
- Foundation Programme: 2 years;
- Anaesthetic Training Programme or Acute Care Common Stem Training (ACCS; 2 years) consisting of 1 year of anaesthesia/intensive care medicine (ICM) and 1 year of acute and emergency medicine. If an ACCS trainee wants to continue in anaesthetic training they will enter year 2 of basic level training;
- Basic level training: 2 years (21 months of anaesthesia and 3 months of ICM);
- Pass the Primary Fellowship of the Royal College of Anaesthetists (FRCA) examination;
- Intermediate level training: 2 years;
- Pass the Final FRCA examination;
- Higher level training: 2 years;
- Advanced level training: 1 year.

Throughout all levels of training, summative assessments are carried out to ensure standards are achieved, with increasing responsibility and the opportunity for subspecialization in the more advanced years of training, for example paediatrics, obstetrics, cardiac, intensive care and pain management.

Useful links

Royal College of Anaesthetists: www.rcoa.ac.uk
Association of Anaesthetists of Great Britain and Ireland: www.aagbi.org

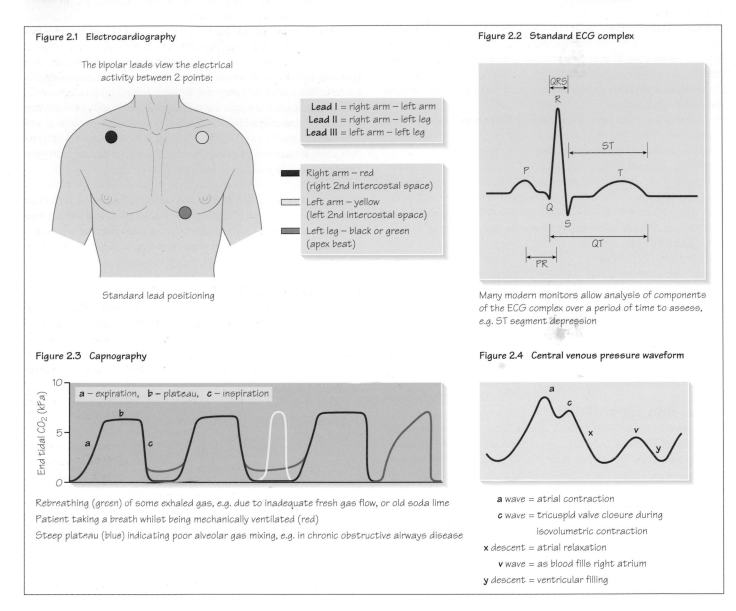

Figure 2.1 Electrocardiography

The bipolar leads view the electrical activity between 2 points:

Lead I = right arm – left arm
Lead II = right arm – left leg
Lead III = left arm – left leg

Right arm – red
(right 2nd intercostal space)
Left arm – yellow
(left 2nd intercostal space)
Left leg – black or green
(apex beat)

Standard lead positioning

Figure 2.2 Standard ECG complex

Many modern monitors allow analysis of components of the ECG complex over a period of time to assess, e.g. ST segment depression

Figure 2.3 Capnography

a – expiration, b – plateau, c – inspiration

End tidal CO_2 (kPa)

Rebreathing (green) of some exhaled gas, e.g. due to inadequate fresh gas flow, or old soda lime
Patient taking a breath whilst being mechanically ventilated (red)
Steep plateau (blue) indicating poor alveolar gas mixing, e.g. in chronic obstructive airways disease

Figure 2.4 Central venous pressure waveform

a wave = atrial contraction
c wave = tricuspid valve closure during isovolumetric contraction
x descent = atrial relaxation
v wave = as blood fills right atrium
y descent = ventricular filling

Routine monitoring can be divided into three categories.

The anaesthetist The anaesthetist is continuously present during the entire administration of an anaesthetic. Information obtained from clinical observation of the patient, monitoring equipment and the progress of the operation allows for the provision of a balanced anaesthetic in terms of: anaesthesia and analgesia, fluid balance, muscle relaxation and general appearance (skin colour, temperature, sweatiness etc.).

The patient The minimum monitoring consists of: electrocardiogram (ECG), pulseoximetry, non-invasive blood pressure, capnography and other gas analysis (O_2, anaesthetic vapour), airway pressure, neuromuscular blockade; see Chapter 12.

The equipment This includes: oxygen analyser, vapour analyser, breathing system, alarms and infusion limits on infusion devices. A means of recording the patient's temperature must be available, as well as a peripheral nerve stimulator when a muscle relaxant is used.

Other monitoring devices are used depending on the type of operation and the medical condition of the patient (e.g. to measure cardiovascular function). These include invasive blood pressure monitoring, central venous pressure, echocardiography, oesophageal Doppler and awareness monitors.

Electrocardiography (ECG)

Continuous assessment of the heart's electrical activity can detect dysrhythmias (lead II) (Figures 2.1 and 2.2) and ischaemia (CM5 position). Most commonly, the standard lead position is used. From this the monitor can be used to measure the electrical activity between two of the leads whilst the third acts as a neutral.

It is important to remember that the heart's electrical activity does not reflect cardiac output or perfusion, for example pulseless electrical

Anaesthesia at a Glance, First Edition. Julian Stone and William Fawcett.

activity (ECG complexes associated with no cardiac output) may be recorded.

Oximetry

A pulse oximeter consists of a light source that emits red and infrared light (650 nm and 805 nm) and a photodetector. The absorption of light at these wavelengths differs in oxygenated and deoxygenated haemoglobin. Thus the relative amount of light detected after passing through a patient's body can be used to estimate the percentage oxygen saturation. The detecting probe is typically placed on the fingernail bed, or ear lobe, and only analyses the pulsatile (arterial) haemoglobin saturation.

Inaccurate readings may be caused by high ambient light levels, poor tissue perfusion (e.g. cardiac failure, hypothermia), cardiac dysrhythmias (e.g. tricuspid regurgitation), nail varnish, methaemoglobinaemia (under reads), carboxyhaemoglobin (over reads) or methylene blue (transient reduction in reading).

There can be a significant delay between an acute event (e.g. apnoea, airway obstruction, disconnection) and a reduction in the S_aO_2 especially if the patient is receiving supplemental oxygen, and any reading should be considered along with other monitoring parameters as well as clinical signs.

Blood pressure (BP) and cardiac output

(Figure 5.4)

A cuff is inflated to above systolic pressure (or to a predetermined figure when taken for the first time in a new patient). A sensing probe detects arterial pulsation at systolic pressure. The maximum amplitude of pulsation is the mean arterial pressure, and the diastolic pressure is derived from the systolic and mean arterial pressures. It is important to be able to measure blood pressure by auscultating the Korotkoff heart sounds. Accurate BP measurement requires an appropriately sized cuff. The width of the cuff should be 20% greater than the diameter of the arm. A large cuff under reads BP, a small cuff over reads.

Care must be taken to avoid soft tissue injury (especially in the elderly) with prolonged periods of use, and nerve entrapment with incorrect cuff placement.

Invasive BP measurement uses an indwelling catheter to measure beat-to-beat variation in BP, and is commonly sited in the radial artery. It has the advantage of recording changes in BP immediately as opposed to non-invasive BP measurement with a cuff, which will only indicate changes in BP when it next cycles.

Indications for invasive BP measurement include: cardiovascular system (CVS) disease (e.g. ischaemic heart disease, valvular heart disease), anticipated instability (e.g. cardiac surgery, operations with large fluid shifts), serial blood samples (e.g. arterial blood gases) in patients who will be going to intensive care postoperatively, and major laparoscopic cases.

Oesophageal Doppler is a non-invasive technique for measuring cardiac output by using ultrasound to measure blood velocity in the descending aorta. This is increasingly used in major operations, especially abdominal surgery.

Gas analysis

The continuous assessment of the gas delivered to and taken from an anaesthetized patient is vital in order to avoid hypoxia and to ensure the delivery of adequate anaesthetic.

Oxygen exhibits paramagnetism, that is it is attracted into an electromagnetic field. The other gases in the sample (CO_2, water vapour, N_2) are diamagnetic and are only weakly affected. The oxygen analyser has two chambers separated by a pressure transducer – a sample chamber and a reference chamber, which contains air. An electromagnetic field is passed through the sample chamber, causing the oxygen present to become agitated. This results in a pressure gradient across the transducer, which is proportional to the partial pressure of oxygen in both chambers. From measurement of this, a percentage oxygen concentration is obtained.

Oxygen failure alarm Nearly all oxygen is delivered via a pipeline and failure of this is very rare. Cylinder oxygen is used when piped gas is not available. A low pressure alarm (independent of an electrical supply) is present on all anaesthetic machines to warn of its failure.

End tidal CO₂ (ETCO₂) monitoring

Extremely useful information is given by monitoring ETCO₂ (capnography; Figure 2.3). Confirmation may be obtained of tracheal intubation, respiratory rate, adequacy of ventilation (i.e. hypo- or hyperventilation), indication of breathing circuit disconnection, indication of sudden circulatory collapse, air embolism and malignant hyperthermia.

Measurement of CO_2 and anaesthetic gases uses infrared absorption spectroscopy. Gases containing at least two different molecules absorb infrared radiation (IR) at specific wavelengths. CO_2 absorbs IR at 4.3 nm. Light is passed through the gas sample continuously and the amount of IR absorbed (recorded by a photodetector) is proportional to the concentration, and therefore partial pressure, of CO_2 and other specific gases such as N_2O and volatile anaesthetics.

The gas sample is most commonly taken as a side-stream from the main breathing circuit (up to 200 mL/min) which can then be returned to the circuit.

Airway pressure

A high pressure alarm is used to help protect the patient from barotrauma (high pressure-related injury).

A low pressure alarm will draw attention to disconnection or apnoea.

Central venous pressure (CVP)

CVP is measured via a large central vein, usually the internal jugular, and provides assessment of the heart's right-sided pressure. The catheter is multilumen and allows measurement of CVP as well as independent fluid administration. It has a characteristic waveform (Figure 2.4).

3 Equipment

Figure 3.1 Anaesthetic equipment

(a) Anaesthetic machine

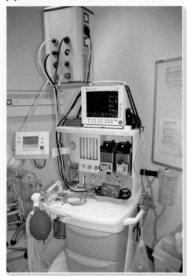

(b) Gas cylinders on the back of the anaesthetic machine (N$_2$O left, O$_2$ right)

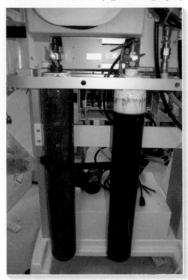

(c) Rotameter

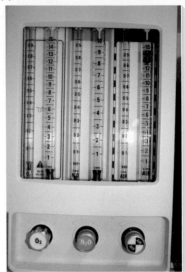

Table 3.1 Cylinder colour — in the UK, cylinders are indentified by the colour of the body and shoulder

Gas		Cylinder body colour	Shoulder colour or pipeline
Oxygen		Black	White
Air		Black	Black/white quarters
Nitrous oxide		French blue	French blue
Entonox		French blue	French blue/white quarters

The majority of gas is supplied by pipeline to anaesthetic machines/ventilators and to wall mounted outlets throughout the hospital. Piped gas is also coloured (see Table 3.1)

Figure 3.2 Bain coaxial circuit

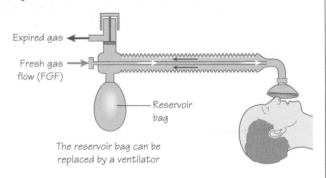

Expired gas

Fresh gas flow (FGF)

Reservoir bag

The reservoir bag can be replaced by a ventilator

Figure 3.3 Circle system

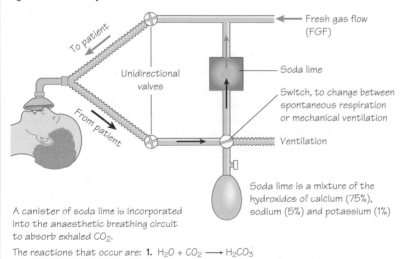

To patient

From patient

Unidirectional valves

Fresh gas flow (FGF)

Soda lime

Switch, to change between spontaneous respiration or mechanical ventilation

Ventilation

Soda lime is a mixture of the hydroxides of calcium (75%), sodium (5%) and potassium (1%)

A canister of soda lime is incorporated into the anaesthetic breathing circuit to absorb exhaled CO_2.

The reactions that occur are:
1. $H_2O + CO_2 \longrightarrow H_2CO_3$
2. $H_2CO_3 + 2\,NaOH \longrightarrow Na_2CO_3 + 2\,H_2O$
3. $Na_2CO_3 + Ca(OH)_2 \longrightarrow CaCO_3 + 2\,NaOH$

Figure 3.4 Laryngoscope blades

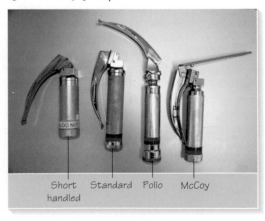

Short handled   Standard   Polio   McCoy

Anaesthesia at a Glance, First Edition. Julian Stone and William Fawcett.

Anaesthetic machine

The anaesthetic machine (Figure 3.1a,b) provides anaesthetic gases in the desired quantities/proportions, at a safe pressure. Gas flow is set on the rotameter (O_2, air, N_2O) (Figure 3.1c), passing to the back bar. Here a proportion (splitting ratio) enters a vaporizer before returning to the main gas flow. The gas leaves the anaesthetic machine at the common gas outlet (CGO), reaching the patient via a breathing circuit.

Vaporizer

Part of the fresh gas flow (FGF) enters the vaporizer. Full saturation with volatile agent is achieved typically by a series of wicks to create a large surface area. As volatile anaesthetic is removed, energy is lost due to latent heat of vaporization. Temperature compensation occurs to maintain output, for example by use of a bimetallic strip which bends as the temperature alters.

Safety features

• **Non-interchangeable screw threads** (NISTs) prevent the incorrect pipeline gas being connected to the machine inlet.
• A **pin index system** is used to prevent incorrect cylinder connection.
• **Barotrauma** to both patient and machine is avoided by using pressure reducing valves/regulators and flow restrictors.
• The **oxygen failure warning alarm** is pressure driven and alerts of imminent pipeline or cylinder failure.
• **Accurate gas delivery:** flow delivered through the anaesthetic machine is displayed by a bobbin (Figure 3.1c) within a rotameter. The gas enters the cylinder at its base, forcing the bobbin higher, depending on the gas flow. This is a fixed pressure, variable orifice flowmeter, that is the pressure difference across the bobbin remains constant whilst the orifice size increases further up the tapered tube. Each rotameter is calibrated for a specific gas as their viscosity (at low, laminar flow) and density (at higher, turbulent flow) affect the height of the bobbin. The bobbins have spiral grooves which cause them to rotate in the gas flow. An antistatic coating prevents the bobbin sticking. Modern anaesthetic machines give a digital representation.
• **Hypoxic guard:** the O_2 and N_2O control knobs are linked, preventing <25% O_2 being delivered when N_2O is used. Oxygen is delivered distal to N_2O within the rotameter, preventing hypoxic gas delivery if the O_2 rotameter is faulty or cracked.
• **Interlocking vaporizers** on the back bar prevent two anaesthetic vapours being given simultaneously.
• **Ventilator alarms** warn of high and low pressure.
• **Emergency oxygen flush:** when pressed, oxygen bypasses the back bar and is delivered to the CGO at >35 L/min. This must be used with caution as gas is delivered at 4 bar and does not contain anaesthetic.
• **Suction:** adjustable negative-pressure-generated suction is used to clear airway secretions/vomit and must be available for all cases.
• **Scavenging** of vented anaesthetic gases is active, passive or a combination. Scavenged gases are usually vented to the atmosphere. Scavenging tubing has a wider bore (30 mm), preventing accidental connection to breathing circuits.

Low gas flows reduce environmental impact and cost. Operating theatre air exchange occurs through the air conditioning system (e.g. 15 times per hour). The main aim is infection control; it also serves to remove unscavenged gases.

Breathing circuits

These deliver the FGF from the CGO to the patient. They are made of corrugated (kink-free) plastic. The FGF is supplied from the anaesthetic machine, wall source or cylinder O_2 (Table 3.1).

An adjustable pressure-limiting (APL) valve is often present. This has a spring-loaded disk that opens at a pressure limit, which can be altered by opening or closing a valve, adding more or less tension to the spring. During assisted ventilation, closure of the valve allows greater inspiratory pressure to be generated before the spill valve opens.

The following are commonly used circuits.

The **Bain circuit** (Figure 3.2) is coaxial. An inner tube leads to the patient (delivering FGF), a surrounding outer tube passes exhaled gas to the anaesthetic machine. It is inefficient during spontaneous breathing as rebreathing of exhaled gas occurs unless the FGF is at least twice the patient's minute volume. It is efficient for controlled ventilation, especially if an expiratory pause occurs, allowing build up of FGF at the patient end of the circuit that is then the first to be delivered with the next inspiration.

A **circle system** (Figure 3.3) allows low FGF during assisted ventilation, and in theory can be only a small amount above the calculated O_2 consumption for the patient (3–4 mL/kg/min for adults, 6–8 mL/kg/min for children). CO_2 is absorbed by soda lime. A higher FGF is needed initially to allow for anaesthetic uptake and nitrogen washout, as well as filling the circuit itself. Within the circle are two one-way valves, an APL valve and a reservoir bag.

Self-inflating bag mask valve has the advantage of not needing an FGF to function, so can work in isolation to deliver room air. It can be connected to an oxygen source; a reservoir bag will further increase inspired O_2 concentration. It incorporates a non-rebreathe valve.

Laryngoscopes

Laryngoscopes are used to visualize the larynx during intubation. The blade is either curved (Macintosh) or straight (Miller) (Figure 3.4). The Macintosh blade is positioned in the vallecula; lifting anteriorly lifts the epiglottis to reveal the larynx. The Miller blade is placed behind the epiglottis and pushes it anteriorly. Examples include:
• The **polio blade** has 135 degree angle between handle and blade and can be used when handle obstruction is encountered, e.g. with obesity.
• The **McCoy blade** has an articulated blade tip. Once the tip is in the vallecula, movement of the tip by pressing a lever on the handle can improve laryngoscopic view.
• **Video laryngoscopes** provide a laryngoscopic view on a screen from a fibre-optic source at the tip of the blade. They have a role in difficult intubations and teaching.
• **Fibre-optic scopes** are used with an endotracheal tube being railroaded over it once the scope is within the trachea.
• A **bougie** is an introducer that can be passed into the larynx (clicks can be felt as the tip passes over tracheal rings) and a tracheal tube is railroaded over it when a poor laryngeal view is seen.

4 Airway devices

Figure 4.1   Guedel airway

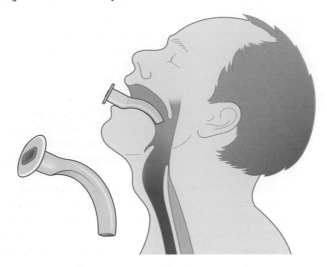

Figure 4.2   Laryngeal face mask: basic type

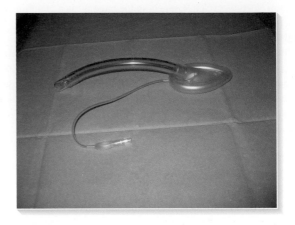

Figure 4.3   Laryngeal mask airway in situ

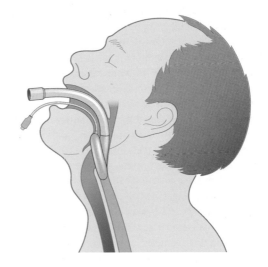

Table 4.1   The laryngeal mask airway (LMA)

Advantages	• Allows hands-free maintenance anaesthesia • Ease of insertion • Can be used by non-anaesthetists • Can be used for difficult/failed tracheal intubation
Disadvantages	• Will not protect against airway soiling • Will not allow ventilation with high airway pressures (high resistance/low compliance) • May become dislodged during anaesthesia

Figure 4.4   Oral tracheal tube (above) and double-lumen tube (below)

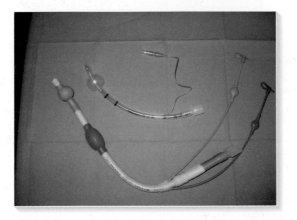

Figure 4.5   Tracheostomy tube

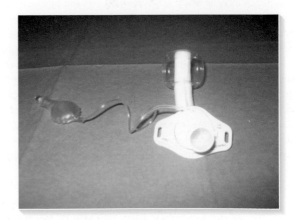

Anaesthesia at a Glance, First Edition. Julian Stone and William Fawcett.

Patients undergoing general anaesthesia or sedation are at risk of both airway obstruction (from relaxation of the musculature supporting the upper airway) and apnoea (caused by respiratory depression and/or paralysis). As oxygen storage in the functional residual capacity in the lungs, even after preoxygenation, is very limited (at most 5 minutes in practice, and in many patients much less), restoring airway patency is the most crucial role for any anaesthetist to undertake. Until the airway is patent, attempts to oxygenate the patient are futile and potentially dangerous as the stomach will probably inflate if the lungs do not (see Chapter 17).

There are a number of devices available and they may be classified according to whether the distal end stops above the vocal cords (supraglottic or extraglottic devices) or passes through the vocal cords (infraglottic or subglottic devices). Prior to insertion, remember it may be possible to restore airway patency by simple manoeuvres such as chin lift and jaw thrust. In addition, remember never to insert your fingers into a patient's mouth and take great care with patients who have loose or crowned teeth.

Supraglottic devices

There have been a large number of devices described in recent years. Many of these (e.g. laryngeal mask airway [LMA, see Figure 4.2]) have been developed not only for their ease of insertion and to maintain the airway, but also to free up the hands of the anaesthetist to perform other tasks.

Simple oral (Guedel) airway

This basic airway device is inserted over the tongue to prevent it falling to the back of the mouth (Figure 4.1). It is available in various sizes from neonates to adults. To judge the correct size, use the distance from the chin to the tragus as a guide. A modification is the cuffed oropharyngeal airway (COPA). This has a distal cuff, which pushes the tongue forward and creates an airtight seal, and the proximal end has a standard 15-mm connector, which is suitable for attachment to an anaesthetic circuit.

Simple nasopharyngeal airway

This soft airway is inserted through the nares and horizontally into the nasopharynx. It is useful when you do not wish to, or are unable to, utilize the patient's mouth. It is tolerated at lighter levels of anaesthesia and also allows suction to the pharynx. However, a major drawback is that haemorrhage may ensue during insertion.

Laryngeal mask airway (Figure 4.2)

Since this device was introduced in the 1980s, it has revolutionized airway management. It frees up the hands of the anaesthetist who, hitherto, had to hold a facemask or intubate the patient's trachea. Initially popularized for spontaneous ventilation, its use has grown to include selected ventilated patients, resuscitation (both in and out of hospital) and in difficult airway algorithms. A summary of its characteristics is shown in Table 4.1.

The original LMA has undergone numerous modifications since it was first developed. When correctly placed it sits over the glottis (Figure 4.3). There are over 25 types available, including:

Flexible LMA This LMA is wire reinforced and is thus less likely to kink. It is particularly useful for head and neck operations when the distal end of the LMA may have an angle of 90 degrees or more.

Intubating LMA This device, once in place, allows the passage of a tracheal tube inside the LMA and past the vocal cords. It is used to allow tracheal intubation when conventional methods have failed.

ProSeal LMA This tube is a newer-generation LMA and has an oesophageal drain tube to permit any GI contents to freely drain out, minimizing the risk of airway soiling. The stomach may also be drained with the insertion of an orogastric tube. In addition, the airway tube is reinforced and the posterior aspect of the cuff increases the seal of the LMA around the laryngeal inlet.

Infraglottic devices

The tip of these devices is positioned below the level of the vocal cords. Unlike the supraglottic devices, they need much more skill at positioning, usually with a laryngoscope, but sometimes they are passed 'blind' or fibre-optically and occasionally under direct vision at a tracheostomy.

The gold standard device is still tracheal intubation, usually with an orotracheal tube (Figure 4.4), but sometimes (especially for intraoral surgery or for fibre-optic intubation) a nasotracheal tube is used (see Chapter 31). Originally made of rubber, they are now usually made of PVC. They usually have a cuff to provide an airtight seal between the tube and the tracheal wall. There are numerous modifications:

RAE (Ring-Adair-Elwyn) tubes These are preformed for head and neck surgery to allow good surgical access. They are commonly used for ENT surgery (see Chapter 31).

Flexometallic (armoured) tubes These are used when positioning of the head may render normal tubes liable to kinking. They are also commonly used for the prone position.

Tubes for ENT surgery (see Chapter 31) These include laser tubes (resistant to laser surgery in the airway and often made of stainless steel), microlaryngeal tubes (small tubes for laryngeal surgery) and tracheostomy (Figure 4.5) and laryngectomy tubes (preformed tubes for insertion directly into the trachea by the surgeon).

Tubes for intensive care These tubes often have high- volume and low- pressure cuffs to protect the tracheal mucosa against long- term damage from the cuff. In addition, they may have a suction port above the cuff to minimize the risk of supraglottic contamination of the airway.

Tubes for thoracic surgery These are generally double-lumen tubes or bronchial blocking tubes to allow differential lung ventilation (see Chapter 21 and Figure 4.4).

Emergency airway devices

These devices are used in order to allow a patent airway when intubation is not possible and especially in the most serious of all airway scenarios 'can't intubate, can't ventilate' (CVCI). The final step in this pathway (following failed mask oxygenation, and LMA insertion) is surgical access to the airway. This involves the use a cannula or direct surgical access via the cricothyroid membrane into the airway. Every anaesthetist should be familiar with the anatomical landmarks of the cricothyroid membrane between the thyroid and cricoid cartilages and the location of cricothyrotomy equipment in theatres.

If time permits, a tracheostomy (Figure 4.5) under local anaesthetic may also be used.

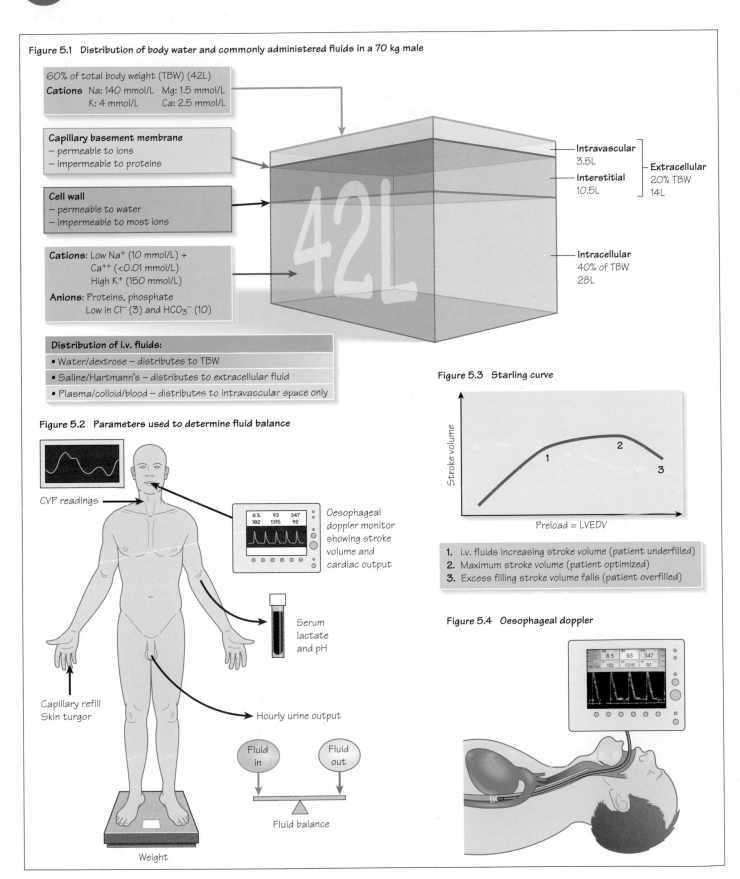

Figure 5.1 Distribution of body water and commonly administered fluids in a 70 kg male

60% of total body weight (TBW) (42L)
Cations Na: 140 mmol/L   Mg: 1.5 mmol/L
K: 4 mmol/L   Ca: 2.5 mmol/L

Capillary basement membrane
– permeable to ions
– impermeable to proteins

Cell wall
– permeable to water
– impermeable to most ions

Cations: Low Na^+ (10 mmol/L) +
Ca^{++} (<0.01 mmol/L)
High K^+ (150 mmol/L)
Anions: Proteins, phosphate
Low in Cl^- (3) and HCO_3^- (10)

Intravascular 3.5L
Interstitial 10.5L — Extracellular 20% TBW 14L
Intracellular 40% of TBW 28L

Distribution of i.v. fluids:
• Water/dextrose – distributes to TBW
• Saline/Hartmann's – distributes to extracellular fluid
• Plasma/colloid/blood – distributes to intravascular space only

Figure 5.2 Parameters used to determine fluid balance

CVP readings

Oesophageal doppler monitor showing stroke volume and cardiac output

Serum lactate and pH

Capillary refill
Skin turgor

Hourly urine output

Fluid in   Fluid out

Fluid balance

Weight

Figure 5.3 Starling curve

Stroke volume
Preload = LVEDV

1. i.v. fluids increasing stroke volume (patient underfilled)
2. Maximum stroke volume (patient optimized)
3. Excess filling stroke volume falls (patient overfilled)

Figure 5.4 Oesophageal doppler

Anaesthesia at a Glance, First Edition. Julian Stone and William Fawcett.

Table 5.1 Oxygen delivery equation – normal values

Oxygen delivery $(DO_2) = CO \times [Hb] \times \%$ oxygen saturation
$\quad (SaO_2) \times 1.34$
$DO_2 = CO \times [Hb] \times 1.34 \times 0.99$
$DO_2 = 5 \times 150 \times 1.34 \times 0.99$
$DO_2 = 1000\,mL\ O_2/min$ approx.

Units: DO_2, mL O_2/min; CO, L/min; Hb, g/L.

Table 5.2 Electrolyte content of various fluids

	Na (mmol/L)	K (mmol/L)	Cl (mmol/L)	HCO$_3$ (mmol/L)	Volume (litres)
Sweat	60	10	45	0	Variable
Gastric juice	60	15	140	0	2–3
Pancreatic juice	130	8	60	85	1–2
Bile	145	5	105	30	0.5

The maintenance of fluid, electrolyte balance and blood volume is crucial to good outcomes following surgery. The fundamental goal is delivery of adequate oxygen to the tissues, which can be expressed by the oxygen delivery equation (Table 5.1) showing the factors that determine oxygen delivery:

- cardiac output (= stroke volume × heart rate);
- haemoglobin concentration;
- oxygen saturation.

Extremes of fluid management have a detrimental outcome, particularly for patients undergoing major surgery and/or patients with poor physiological reserve. Too little fluid results in dehydration and haemoconcentration, leading to a poor cardiac output and oxygen delivery to the tissues. If left untreated, in the early stages compensation will occur with increased oxygen extraction and a switch to anaerobic metabolism and production of lactic acid. Eventually, there will be organ failure when compensatory mechanisms are exhausted. Conversely, excess fluid management will overwhelm the circulation, with fluid will leaking out into the tissues, causing oedema. This too will impede cellular oxygenation and healing and causes organ dysfunction, especially in the lungs. For many patients there may be a considerable amount of physiological reserve and they may cope well with relative extremes of fluid balance, but for some patients the margins between inadequate and excessive fluid administration may be very small.

Fluid compartments

The body contains approximately 60% water. Approximately two-thirds of this is intracellular, and one-third extracellular, with the extracellular fluid further subdivided into interstitial and intravascular fluid. Figure 5.1 shows these compartments. There are two points to note:

1 There are marked differences in biochemistry between intracellular and extracellular compartments. Intracellular fluid is rich in potassium and fixed anions (protein, phosphate and sulphate). Extracellular fluid is rich in sodium and chloride and low in potassium. Thus serum estimation is a good representative of total body sodium but unreliable for total body potassium.
2 There are two compartmental divisions:
   (a) cell membrane, which is permeable to water but impermeable to most ions except via channels, e.g. Na/K pump;
   (b) capillary basement membrane, which is impermeable to most proteins but permeable to ions.

Knowledge of these two membranes enables us to deduce the volume of distribution of administered i.v. fluids.

Intravenous fluids

There are various types of fluid available for administration to patients:

Dextrose Dextrose is metabolized leaving the water, which distributes freely within the total body water. Therefore, for every 1 litre of dextrose administered i.v. only a little over 100 mL will remain in the vascular compartment. Large quantities will cause hyperglycaemia and dilutional hyponatraemia.

Crystalloids These solutions contain electrolytes in a similar concentration to extracellular fluid. Hartmann's solution is most similar to extracellular fluid (although it contains lactate rather than bicarbonate). They will distribute within the extravascular compartment but not within the intracellular compartment (as the cell membrane prevents free transfer of electrolytes). Hence, for every 1 litre of saline administered i.v. only approximately 250 mL will remain in the vascular compartment. Hartmann's solution is the traditional crystalloid for use in theatres. Excessive saline can cause a hyperchloraemic alkalosis.

Colloids These are suspensions of osmotically active, large particles. They are usually of either starch or gelatin in origin. Initially, they are largely confined to the vascular compartment, although some have only a relatively short half-life prior to excretion.

Blood and blood products These (e.g. albumen, fresh frozen plasma) are also confined to the intravascular compartment.

Fluid prescribing

In calculating appropriate fluid balance, the following need to be taken into account:

1 maintenance requirements;
2 perioperative losses;
   (a) preoperative;
   (b) peroperative;
   (c) postoperative.

For maintenance of fluids, adult patients should receive sodium 50–100 mmol/day and potassium 40–80 mmol/day in approx 2.5 litres of water by the oral, enteral or parenteral route. To replace other losses, the estimation must include both the volume and electrolyte content of the fluid (Table 5.2). In addition, particularly for rapid infusions (e.g. during haemorrhage), it should be recognize that there will be dilution of other constituents of the vascular compartment, most importantly red cells, platelets and clotting factors.

Assessment of fluid status

The aim of fluid management is to ensure that the patient's fluid status is optimized. This is particularly important prior to emergency surgery.

There are many indicators that can assist in this process, as shown in Figure 5.2. Weight is a simple and underused measurement, useful in monitoring over several days. In theory, fluid balance charts (e.g. input/output charts) should be useful but in practice may be inaccurate or incomplete. Skin turgor and capillary refill may be useful when dehydration is marked but may be affected by other causes such as cachexia and old age.

Urine output is a useful indicator of fluid balance and will require a urinary catheter and hourly measurements to be undertaken accurately. However, there are other factors here: diuretics will dramatically increase urine output and conversely major surgery will reduce urine output. Usually, 0.5 mL/kg/h (or 30 mL/h in total) is considered the minimum required volume.

Pulse and blood pressure may both indicate that the patient is hypovolaemic, although blood pressure in particular may remain normal until the process is advanced. Central venous pressure (CVP) is often used to guide therapy for these patients. The normal central venous pressure is 4–8 mmHg, and is an indicator of right ventricular end diastolic pressure (RVEDP). There is an assumption that this will reflect left ventricular end diastolic pressure (LVEDP) and indeed left ventricular end diastolic volume (LVEDV). This latter measurement is effectively cardiac preload. There are clearly a number of assumptions from CVP to LVEDV, including compliance (stiffness) of the heart but it is nevertheless a technique that is commonly used to guide fluid balance.

The fundamental process of the heart responding to stretching (i.e. fluid challenge) by increasing its stroke volume is the clinical application of Starling's Law, whereby stretching of heart fibres produces an increased force of contraction (Figure 5.3). However, excessive stretching will exhaust this process, causing the heart to fail, and so a key area is to find the optimum filling of the heart but avoid overfilling, which will cause the force of contraction and stroke volume to decline again. Patients are given a bolus of fluid (e.g. 250 mL of colloid) and if the stroke volume significantly increases the process is repeated until the stroke volume no longer rises. This is taken to be the point at which the patient's fluid status is optimized.

Recently, whilst both pressure measurements (e.g. CVP) and flow measurements (e.g. stroke volume) are considered to be important, the use of flow measurements (e.g. oesophageal Doppler) to guide fluid management is increasing (Figure 5.4).

Finally, various biochemical markers are used but there may be a delay of several hours for these to respond to changes. They include lactate and pH measurements from arterial blood gas analysis.

Finding the balance between inadequate and excess fluid administration is not easy, particularly in those with limited reserve. A key point is the way in which a patient's urine output, CVP or stroke volume responds to a fluid challenge. Careful assessment of this response, and repeating it if appropriate, is the cornerstone to optimizing a patient's fluid status.

Table 6.1 NCEPOD classification of intervention

	Description	Example
Immediate	• Life/limb/organ saving • Resuscitation occurs simultaneously with surgery • Surgery within minutes	Rapid bleeding, e.g. trauma, aneurysm
Urgent	• Life/limb/organ threatening • Surgery within hours	Perforated bowel or less urgent bleeding
Expedited	• Early surgery (within a day or two)	Large bowel obstruction, closed long bone fracture
Elective	• Timing to suit patient and hospital	Joint replacement, unobstructed hernia repair, cataract

Table 6.2 Surgical factors in assessment of risk of significant cardiac event

Low risk <1%	• Minor orthopaedic and urology • Gynaecology • Breast • Dental
Intermediate 1–5%	• Major orthopaedic and urology • Abdominal • Head and neck
High risk >5%	• Aortic, major vascular • Peripheral vascular • Intraperitoneal/intrathoracic

Figure 6.1 Patient factors associated with cardiac risk

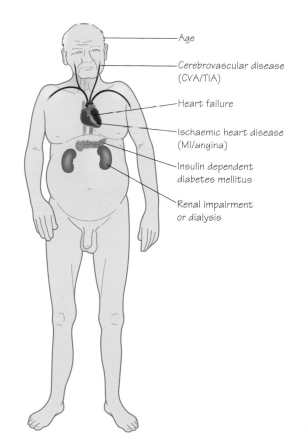

Age

Cerebrovascular disease (CVA/TIA)

Heart failure

Ischaemic heart disease (MI/angina)

Insulin dependent diabetes mellitus

Renal impairment or dialysis

Figure 6.2 Patients at risk of gastric aspiration even after fasting

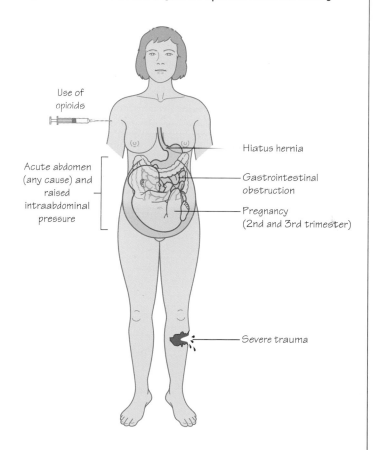

Use of opioids

Hiatus hernia

Acute abdomen (any cause) and raised intraabdominal pressure

Gastrointestinal obstruction

Pregnancy (2nd and 3rd trimester)

Severe trauma

Anaesthesia at a Glance, First Edition. Julian Stone and William Fawcett.
© 2013 Julian Stone and William Fawcett. Published 2013 by John Wiley & Sons, Ltd. **21**

There are a number of issues to consider in preparing the patient for surgery, including the timing of surgery, improving the physical status of the patient, information for the patient and ensuring that the correct procedure is carried out.

Timing of surgery

There are various classifications of the urgency of surgery; the most common is the NCEPOD classification (National Confidential Enquiry into Patient Outcome and Death), given in Table 6.1. The anaesthetist has to ensure that the patient is made as well as they can be made prior to surgery. In immediate cases, there will be no time to effect improvement in the patient's condition beforehand, as resuscitation takes place simultaneously during surgery. Fortunately such cases are quite rare; with most 'emergencies' there are a few hours which can be well spent to reduce risk and improve outcome by careful treatment (vascular access, urinary catheter, nasogastric tube, i.v. fluids). With elective patients there is plenty of time to make the patient as well as they can be (e.g. treatment of hypertension or angina). In some cases it may be appropriate to refer the patients for other surgery first (e.g. coronary revascularization or carotid surgery prior to, for example, a joint replacement).

Assessment of risk

Patients may ask about the risks associated with their procedure. Whilst it is not possible to give an exact figure, there are two main areas to consider – the patient (Figures 6.1) and the proposed surgery (Table 6.2). Cardiac risk is the major area that has been studied, as perioperative cardiac events are not uncommon and carry a significant mortality.

There are many general risk-scoring systems; the most well known is the American Society of Anesthesiologists (ASA) grading (Table 6.3), but there are many others including POSSUM (Physiological and Operative Severity Score for enUMeration of morbidity and mortality), APACHE (Acute Physiology and Chronic Health Evaluation) and various others specifically for cardiac risk such the Goldman (1977) and Lee's modification of this in 1999.

Table 6.3 ASA grading

ASA grade	Definition	Example
I	A normal healthy patient	
II	A patient with mild systemic disease	Well-controlled hypertension, asthma
III	A patient with severe systemic disease	Controlled CHF, stable angina
IV	A patient with severe systemic disease that is a constant threat to life	Unstable angina, symptomatic COPD, symptomatic CHF
V	A moribund patient who is not expected to survive without the operation	Multiorgan failure, sepsis syndrome with haemodynamic instability
VI	A declared brain-dead patient whose organs are being removed for donor purposes	

Emergencies are followed by the letter E.
CHF, congestive heart failure; COPD, chronic obstructive pulmonary disease.

Unsurprisingly, sick and/or elderly patients with significant co-morbidities tolerate major surgery poorly (especially emergency surgery).

Preoperative assessment clinics

The vast majority of patients are admitted on the day of surgery. It is then too late to order further tests and therefore, unless problems are picked up in advance of the admission, cancellation rates will be unacceptably high. Therefore, once scheduled for surgery, patients attend a preassessment clinic to identify, and if necessary treat, co-morbidities in attempt to reduce complications. There are a number of areas involved in this process.

History and examination

The general medical assessment includes:
- cardiac disease, e.g. angina, hypertension, myocardial ischaemia, heart failure, valvular disease;
- respiratory disease, e.g. chronic obstructive pulmonary disease (COPD), asthma, infection;
- GI disease, e.g. reflux, liver disease;
- renal disease, e.g. renal impairment;
- CNS disease, e.g. transient ischaemic attack (TIA), cerebrovascular accident (CVA);
- musculoskeletal disease, e.g. rheumatoid arthritis;
- endocrine disease, e.g. diabetes;
- medication, including non-prescription drugs and herbal remedies;
- allergies;
- tobacco, alcohol and recreational drugs.

In addition, there are areas specifically related to anaesthesia.
- **The airway**: in order to undertake tracheal intubation (which may be required in any patient) you will need to take a history and examine the airway. From the history, documented difficulties with airway management, cervical spine problems (e.g. previous surgery or ankylosis), trauma or infection to the airway, previous scarring of the head and neck (e.g. radiotherapy or burns) and temporomandibular joint dysfunction all suggest potential problems with tracheal intubation. On examination, poor mouth opening, obesity, a receding mandible and inability to protrude the mandible also suggest that tracheal intubation may be difficult.
- **Past anaesthetic history**: ask specifically about anaesthetic problems.
- **Family history**: ask specifically about malignant hyperthermia.

Preoperative tests

Common tests include full blood count, electrolytes and urea, coagulation screen, ECG and chest X ray. In recent years, the emphasis has been on targeting tests to those at risk of abnormality, where either knowledge of the abnormalities would change management (e.g. investigation or treatment of anaemia) or act as a baseline for likely changes (e.g. ECG and chest X ray for cardiothoracic surgery). There is very little value in screening healthy patients with a battery of tests. However, urinalysis should be carried out for all patients.

For patients at risk and/or those undergoing major surgery (particularly vascular surgery) further, more detailed tests might include:
- liver function tests;
- arterial blood gas analysis;
- respiratory function tests;
- cardiac echocardiography and other imaging (including angiography) to assess left ventricular function, valve gradients and quantify ischaemic heart disease;

• cervical spine X ray may be required in those with suspected cervical spine degeneration, surgery and trauma as neck mobility is a key determinant of ease of tracheal intubation.

The final focus of preoperative tests involves the degree of physiological reserve and there are various tests to quantify this, such as cardiopulmonary exercise testing (CPET).

Perioperative medication

Generally, all medication is continued perioperatively except:
• drugs that affect coagulation (warfarin, heparin, aspirin, clopidogrel);
• hypoglycaemics;
• some hypotensive drugs, e.g. ACE inhibitors are stopped only on the day of surgery.

For drugs that affect coagulation the relative risk of stopping the drug (thromboembolism) or continuing (perioperative bleeding) has to be ascertained. In some circumstances the drugs are omitted altogether, or the patient transferred to a low dose or therapeutic doses of low-molecular-weight heparin. For insulin-dependent diabetic patients, long-acting insulin is generally discontinued and a sliding scale with short-acting i.v. insulin is commenced (see Chapter 29).

In addition, some drugs may be commenced in the preoperative period, such as β blockers, ACE inhibitors or statins, to further reduce risk.

Fasting

No anaesthetic should be undertaken (unless it is an emergency) until the patient is fasted. This is to prevent both gastric acid and particulate matter entering the tracheobronchial tree, which can cause in the former case pneumonitis and in the latter case airway obstruction. Therefore elective surgery should not proceed unless the patient has had >2 hours since clear fluid, >4 hours since milk and >6 hours since food.

However, there are patients in whom the stomach can never guaranteed to be empty and these are shown in Figure 6.2. These patients are at risk of aspiration of gastric contents and will require early tracheal intubation to protect the airway.

Preoperative care

The ward staff will prepare and ensure the patient is ready for theatre. Deep venous thrombosis (DVT) prophylaxis, methicillin resistant *Staphylococcus aureus* testing, together with all the preassessment paperwork, are collated.

The anaesthetist should always see the patient on the ward prior to arrival in theatre. A consultation in the anaesthetic room is unacceptable – the patient has no time to take on board the information, discuss with family or friends and will feel pressured to comply. A full check of all preassessment details is undertaken and the results of any tests reviewed.

Arrival in theatre

The patient will be checked in and anaesthesia commenced. Once in theatre, the WHO checklist (see Figure 8.2) will again check the patient, procedure and address specific concerns such as blood loss, glycaemic control and antibiotic prophylaxis with anaesthetists, surgeons and nursing staff, all ensuring that they are happy with their responsibilities.

Figure 7.1 The four ways heat is lost

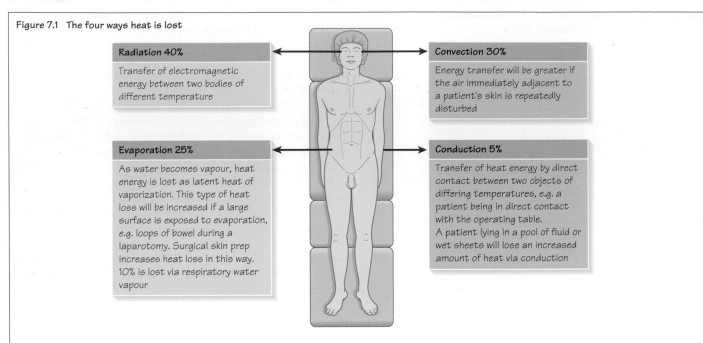

Radiation 40%

Transfer of electromagnetic energy between two bodies of different temperature

Convection 30%

Energy transfer will be greater if the air immediately adjacent to a patient's skin is repeatedly disturbed

Evaporation 25%

As water becomes vapour, heat energy is lost as latent heat of vaporization. This type of heat loss will be increased if a large surface is exposed to evaporation, e.g. loops of bowel during a laparotomy. Surgical skin prep increases heat loss in this way. 10% is lost via respiratory water vapour

Conduction 5%

Transfer of heat energy by direct contact between two objects of differing temperatures, e.g. a patient being in direct contact with the operating table.
A patient lying in a pool of fluid or wet sheets will lose an increased amount of heat via conduction

Figure 7.2 The three phases of heat loss during anaesthesia

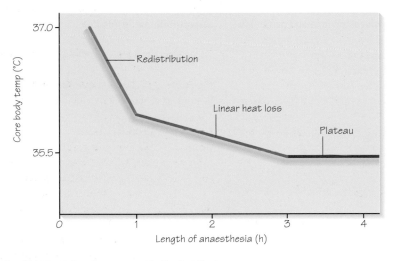

Redistribution

Linear heat loss

Plateau

Figure 7.3 Methods to maintain temperature in an anaesthetized patient

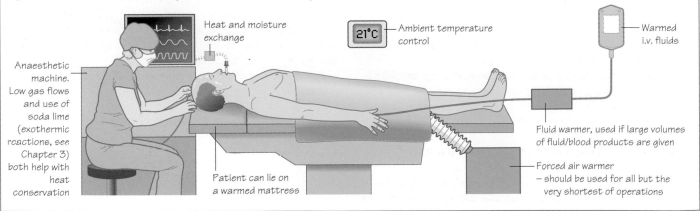

Heat and moisture exchange

Ambient temperature control

Warmed i.v. fluids

Anaesthetic machine. Low gas flows and use of soda lime (exothermic reactions, see Chapter 3) both help with heat conservation

Patient can lie on a warmed mattress

Fluid warmer, used if large volumes of fluid/blood products are given

Forced air warmer – should be used for all but the very shortest of operations

Anaesthesia at a Glance, First Edition. Julian Stone and William Fawcett.

Patients lose heat during the perioperative period. Heat loss can start on the ward or during transfer to the theatre suite, especially if wearing only a thin theatre gown. It is more common in children, especially babies, as they have a larger surface area to body mass ratio.

Hypothermia in this setting is defined as a core temperature <36.0°C. If a patient's preoperative temperature is <36°C then active warming measures should be instituted. Anaesthesia should be delayed for elective cases until the temperature is >36°C.

The body loses heat in four ways: **radiation**, **convection**, **evaporation** and **conduction** (Figure 7.1).

Afferent information is conducted from the skin's thermoreceptors (hot and cold) to the anterior hypothalamus. Efferent responses are relayed via the posterior hypothalamus.

Autonomic control of temperature is mediated by:
- shivering;
- non-shivering thermogenesis, which occurs in brown adipose tissue (sympathetic); a large amount exists in neonates but only a small amount in adults, where it contributes <10–15% of heat production;
- sweating;
- changes in peripheral vascular smooth muscle tone.

Factors contributing to heat loss during anaesthesia are:
- alteration of autonomic control;
- peripheral vasodilatation, e.g. by volatile anaesthetics;
- use of surgical skin prep;
- exposed surgical site (e.g. laparotomy);
- removal of behavioural responses, e.g. clothes etc.;
- poor nutritional status/thin patients with a paucity of insulating fat.

Effect of anaesthesia on temperature control Central control within the hypothalamus is altered so that heat-conserving measures are triggered at a lower temperature and heat-losing processes are initiated at a higher temperature. Impairment of thermoregulatory responses causes three phases of heat loss during anaesthesia (Figure 7.2):
Phase 1: Redistribution – initial rapid heat redistribution from core to periphery. There is no net loss of total body heat during the 1st hour.
Phase 2: Linear – a slower continued heat loss. Heat loss is greater than metabolic heat production in the subsequent 2 hours.
Phase 3: Plateau – heat production equals heat loss after 3 hours.

Consequences of hypothermia

The consequences of hypothermia are:
- shivering, with increased O_2 consumption/increased CO_2 production;
- impaired white cell function leading to postoperative infection;
- impaired platelet function leading to postoperative bleeding/haematomas;
- altered drug metabolism.

All the above may cause delayed recovery from surgery and therefore delayed discharge home.

It is important to avoid patients overheating during anaesthesia. Patients who are being actively warmed during anaesthesia need temperature monitoring. This is to assess the effectiveness of the warming method as well as to avoid overheating.

Monitoring temperature during anaesthesia

Ways of measuring temperature interoperatively are:
- infrared tympanic thermometer, which measures infrared radiation from the tympanic membrane; it is simple to use and a rapid reading is given;
- nasopharyngeal or oesophageal thermistor;
- thermistor within the pulmonary artery (e.g. within a pulmonary artery catheter);
- liquid crystal thermometer – heat sensitive crystals in a plastic strip which can be applied to the forehead;

A thermistor is a semiconductor whose electrical resistance falls as temperature increases; it responds rapidly to changes in temperature.

Maintaining temperature during anaesthesia (Figure 7.3)

Warmed/humidified gases A heat and moisture exchange filter is usually incorporated into the breathing circuit. This absorbs heat and water vapour from exhaled respiratory gases and helps warm and humidify the next delivery of gases to the patient. It is not as effective as active warming methods.

Forced air warmer This blows warm air into a double-layered sheet that covers as much of the patient as possible.

Fluid warmer/warmed fluids If >500 mL of fluid is given it should be warmed to 37°C using a fluid warmer, as should all blood products.

Warmed blankets
Simple and effective for short cases.

Ambient temperature In modern operating theatres temperature can be accurately controlled and should be at least 21°C.

Silver-lined space blankets/hats These reduce radiation heat loss.

Postoperative shivering

Postoperative shivering can occur due to:
- hypothermia;
- general anaesthesia itself;
- regional anaesthesia (e.g. spinal or epidural anaesthesia).

Shivering can be unpleasant, especially if movement exacerbates pain. It increases oxygen consumption, which can lead to inadequate oxygen provision to other essential organs. This could result in cerebral ischaemia (can present with confusion) or myocardial ischaemia (e.g. angina, cardiac failure, dysrhythmias).

In non-shivering thermogenesis, uncoupling of oxidative phosphorylation occurs with the production of heat energy instead of adenosine triphosphate. It is more important in neonatal heat production, and is mediated via the sympathetic nervous system (β3 receptors).

Routine recovery room monitoring (non-invasive blood pressure, saturation monitor, ECG) can be affected by shivering or other movement.

Drugs that can be used to avoid or treat shivering include:
- pethidine
- ondansetron
- anticholinesterases, e.g. physostigmine
- propofol
- doxapram.

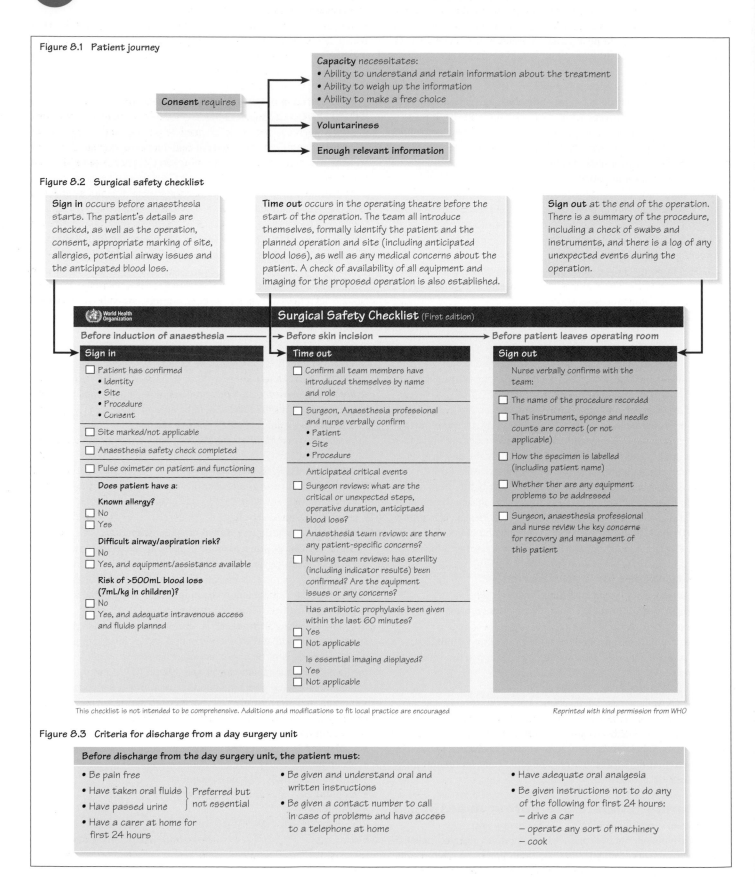

Figure 8.1 Patient journey

Consent requires →

Capacity necessitates:
- Ability to understand and retain information about the treatment
- Ability to weigh up the information
- Ability to make a free choice

Voluntariness

Enough relevant information

Figure 8.2 Surgical safety checklist

Sign in occurs before anaesthesia starts. The patient's details are checked, as well as the operation, consent, appropriate marking of site, allergies, potential airway issues and the anticipated blood loss.

Time out occurs in the operating theatre before the start of the operation. The team all introduce themselves, formally identify the patient and the planned operation and site (including anticipated blood loss), as well as any medical concerns about the patient. A check of availability of all equipment and imaging for the proposed operation is also established.

Sign out at the end of the operation. There is a summary of the procedure, including a check of swabs and instruments, and there is a log of any unexpected events during the operation.

World Health Organization

Surgical Safety Checklist (First edition)

Before induction of anaesthesia —————→ Before skin incision ————————→ Before patient leaves operating room

Sign in

- [ ] Patient has confirmed
  - Identity
  - Site
  - Procedure
  - Consent

- [ ] Site marked/not applicable

- [ ] Anaesthesia safety check completed

- [ ] Pulse oximeter on patient and functioning

Does patient have a:

Known allergy?
- [ ] No
- [ ] Yes

Difficult airway/aspiration risk?
- [ ] No
- [ ] Yes, and equipment/assistance available

Risk of >500mL blood loss (7mL/kg in children)?
- [ ] No
- [ ] Yes, and adequate intravenous access and fluids planned

Time out

- [ ] Confirm all team members have introduced themselves by name and role

- [ ] Surgeon, Anaesthesia professional and nurse verbally confirm
  - Patient
  - Site
  - Procedure

Anticipated critical events

- [ ] Surgeon reviews: what are the critical or unexpected steps, operative duration, anticiptaed blood loss?

- [ ] Anaesthesia team reviews: are therw any patient-specific concerns?

- [ ] Nursing team reviews: has sterility (including indicator results) been confirmed? Are the equipment issues or any concerns?

Has antibiotic prophylaxis been given within the last 60 minutes?
- [ ] Yes
- [ ] Not applicable

Is essential imaging displayed?
- [ ] Yes
- [ ] Not applicable

Sign out

Nurse verbally confirms with the team:

- [ ] The name of the procedure recorded

- [ ] That instrument, sponge and needle counts are correct (or not applicable)

- [ ] How the specimen is labelled (including patient name)

- [ ] Whether ther are any equipment problems to be addressed

- [ ] Surgeon, anaesthesia professional and nurse review the key concerns for recovery and management of this patient

This checklist is not intended to be comprehensive. Additions and modifications to fit local practice are encouraged

Reprinted with kind permission from WHO

Figure 8.3 Criteria for discharge from a day surgery unit

Before discharge from the day surgery unit, the patient must:

- Be pain free
- Have taken oral fluids } Preferred but
- Have passed urine } not essential
- Have a carer at home for first 24 hours

- Be given and understand oral and written instructions
- Be given a contact number to call in case of problems and have access to a telephone at home

- Have adequate oral analgesia
- Be given instructions not to do any of the following for first 24 hours:
  – drive a car
  – operate any sort of machinery
  – cook

Anaesthesia at a Glance, First Edition. Julian Stone and William Fawcett.

Preoperative stage

Once a patient is listed for a particular operation, they follow a series of steps. Patients attend a preoperative assessment clinic, which will be nurse-led for low-risk patients and doctor-led for higher-risk patients who have co-morbidities (e.g. cardiovascular or respiratory disease). Questionnaires filled out in advance identify patients needing to attend the doctor-led clinic.

Those identified as at high-risk for anaesthesia/surgery due to their premorbid state will ideally attend an anaesthetic clinic. Here they will be assessed and examined by an anaesthetist and specialist investigations arranged, including:

* echocardiography;
* lung function tests;
* cardiopulmonary exercise testing;
* coronary angiography;
* routine investigations will already have been arranged, depending on the patient's age, sex and general health:
  * blood tests (haematology, biochemistry)
  * chest X ray
  * ECG.

Patients who have not been seen in an assessment will be seen by the anaesthetist either the evening before or, increasingly often, on the day of surgery.

Anaesthetic consent is an important aspect of operative consent. All patients should have received written information in advance (see Figure 8.1 for a summary of the components of consent). Patients should have the opportunity to discuss options for the type of anaesthesia (e.g. local vs. general) as well as an explanation of side effects:

* common side effects, e.g. postoperative nausea and vomiting (PONV; see Chapter 14);
* rare side effects, e.g. nerve damage after spinal or epidural anaesthesia;
* risks specific to that patient – this can relate to a career (e.g. an opera singer and the risk of vocal cord injury) or the risk of perioperative myocardial infarction in a patient with a significant history of cardiac disease.

Consent must be obtained before any sedating premedication is given. It is important to clearly document the information discussed during consent. Some countries (but not the UK) require a signed anaesthetic consent form.

When a patient's operation is due, they are transferred from the ward to the anaesthetic room or operating theatre. This can be directly or via a holding bay where patients wait until their operation is due. They will often walk, or will be transferred on a trolley or in a wheelchair if unable to do so due to, for example, disability or sedative premedication.

Intraoperative stage

The patient arrives in the anaesthetic room, if this is used. This is normal practice in the UK but they do not exist in North America. In other countries (e.g. New Zealand) they are used briefly to establish i.v. access and apply monitoring before moving into the operating theatre.

Monitoring is applied, including ECG, pulse oximeter, non-invasive blood pressure. Other monitoring might be used at this stage depending on the clinical state of the patient (e.g. invasive blood pressure monitoring).

Intravenous access is established. A small cannula is used if minimal blood loss is anticipated. A larger-bore cannula will be sited in situations where fluid replacement may need to be given quickly or in situations where blood and blood products may need to be given. This can be inserted once the patient is anaesthetized or before induction, using local anaesthetic to the skin beforehand.

Patients may have interventions before undergoing general anaesthesia. These are often performed at this stage, allowing the patient to draw attention to paraesthesia or pain, and include:

* spinal or epidural insertion;
* peripheral nerve blocks.

After induction of anaesthesia, the patient's airway is secured (e.g. with an LMA or endotracheal tube). Once this is complete any further monitoring/interventions are performed (e.g. insertion of an oral or nasogastric tube, central venous cannula, oesophageal Doppler). Application of limb tourniquets and urinary catheter insertion occur, if indicated.

The patient is transiently disconnected from all monitoring and anaesthetic gas source and transferred to the adjacent operating theatre. Here, they are transferred onto the operating table, unless they are already on one, or a patient trolley that can be used for operating.

The World Health Organization (WHO) have introduced a checklist (Figure 8.2) to be completed before the start of operations, in order to reduce morbidity from factors such as surgery at the wrong site, omission of intraoperative antibiotics and thromboprophylaxis. The need for active patient warming and blood sugar control is also discussed by theatre staff.

Postoperative stage

At the end of the operation, the patient is either extubated in the operating theatre (and an oropharyngeal airway inserted if needed) or transferred to the recovery room with an LMA still *in situ*. All patients receive supplemental oxygen during transfer.

Many patients who do not have a general anaesthetic/sedation bypass the recovery room and go straight from the operating theatre to stage 2 recovery in the day surgery unit. Examples include local anaesthetic cases (e.g. minor surface surgery, cataract removal, some regional anaesthetic cases).

Once in the recovery room, a handover occurs between the anaesthetist and a recovery nurse. Important information passed on includes:

* patients name and age;
* operation details;
* blood loss;
* anaesthetic technique with emphasis on:
  * analgesia given;
  * regional/nerve blocks;
  * antiemetics given;
  * antibiotics;
  * the use of local anaesthetic infiltration;
  * thromboprophylaxis.

Further analgesia is given if needed, including management of epidurals, as well as antiemetics and fluids. Patients stay in the recovery room until they are:

* awake and in complete control of airway reflexes;
* pain free;
* no/minimal nausea and vomiting;
* no/minimal bleeding from surgical site;
* normothermic.

Once discharged from the recovery room, patients return to the ward if they are an inpatient or to stage 2 recovery for day surgery patients. Patients must meet certain criteria before they are discharged (Figure 8.3).

9 General anaesthesia – inhalational anaesthetics

Table 9.1 Properties of commonly used agents

	Molecular weight (MW)	Minimum alveolar concentration	Blood/gas coefficient	Oil/gas coefficient	% Metabolized
Nitrous oxide	44	104	0.47	1.4	–
Isoflurane	184.5	1.15	1.43	91	2
Sevoflurane	200	2	0.69	53	5
Desflurane	168	6.35	0.42	19	0.02
Halothane	1974	0.75	2.4	224	20

Table 9.2 Factors affecting minimum alveolar concentration (MAC)

MAC ↓   Age (peak at 6 months)
Premedication (e.g. benzodiazepines)
Opioids
Pregnancy
Acute alcohol intoxication
Other volatiles (MACs are additive. 0.6 of one agent + 0.4 of another = 1 MAC)
Nitrous oxide
Hypothermia
MAC ↑   Chronic alcohol consumption (liver enzyme induction)
Increased sympathetic activity (e.g. amphetamine, cocaine)
Hypermetabolic states (e.g. thyrotoxicosis, pyrexia)
Anxiety
Some antidepressants (tricyclics, monoamine oxidase inhibitors)

Table 9.3 Properties of the ideal volatile anaesthetic agent

Non-toxic
Non-allergenic
Not a malignant hyperthermia (MH) trigger
Stable in storage, non-flammable
No extra specialist equipment needed
Low blood/gas coefficient
Low oil/gas coefficient
Analgesic
CVS stable
No respiratory depression
Non-irritant
Not metabolized
Environmentally inert
Expensive
No reaction with soda lime/breathing circuit

Figure 9.1 Anaesthetic gases

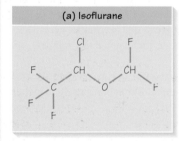

(a) Isoflurane

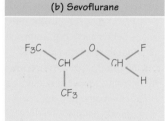

(b) Sevoflurane

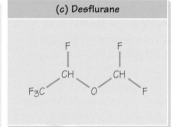

(c) Desflurane

(d) Halothane

Volatile anaesthetics are liquids at room temperature. Part of the FGF passes through a vaporizer on the anaesthetic machine, becoming fully saturated with the vaporizer's agent; it is then returned to the FGF. This gaseous form is inhaled by the patient, maintaining anaesthesia. In certain circumstances inhalational agents can be used to induce anaesthesia (e.g. children, difficult i.v. access, difficult intubation, upper airway obstruction).

The main volatile agents currently used are isoflurane, sevoflurane and desflurane. All are halogenated ethers, their properties depending on the specific halogenation. The mechanism of action is still not fully understood but key points include:
• action at pre- and/or postsynaptic ligand-gated channels – lipophilic sites;
• interruption of information processing and memory establishment;

• potentiation of inhibitory effect of γ-aminobutyric acid (GABA) at $GABA_A$ receptors;
• inhibition of transmission at excitatory N-methyl-D-aspartate (NMDA) receptors.

The potency of a volatile anaesthetic is related to its lipid solubility –the more lipophilic, the greater its potency. This is expressed as the oil/gas solubility coefficient.

The blood/gas solubility coefficient describes the rate of uptake of the agent and the speed with which adequate partial pressure of the agent is exerted within brain tissues to induce and/or maintain anaesthesia –the lower the coefficient, the quicker a steady state is reached; the greater the coefficient, the longer it takes for equilibrium of partial pressures between the alveoli and brain tissue to be met, and hence a slower speed of on- and offset (Table 9.1).

Anaesthesia at a Glance, First Edition. Julian Stone and William Fawcett.

Minimum alveolar concentration (MAC)

Each agent has a specific minimum alveolar concentration (MAC), defined as *the amount of vapour (%) needed to render 50% of spontaneously breathing patients unresponsive to a standard painful surgical stimulus.* MAC is inversely proportional to potency. See Table 9.2 for factors affecting MAC.

General effects

CNS Many agents produce a dose-dependent reduction in cerebral activity (represented as a reduction in level of consciousness and EEG activity). Oxygen consumption is reduced and cerebral blood flow (and intracranial pressure) increases.

RS Many agents cause reduced alveolar minute ventilation by reduced tidal volume and increased respiratory rate. Respiratory response to hypoxia and hypercarbia is reduced.

CVS Many agents cause myocardial depression by reducing myocardial contractility; they reduce systemic vascular resistance and change heart rate. All produce a net hypotensive effect.

Skeletal muscle There is reduced muscle tone and potentiation of muscle relaxants.

Basal metabolic rate This is reduced; a MAC of 2 reduces oxygen consumption by 30%.

Isoflurane (Figure 9.1(a))

Isoflurane causes a drop in blood pressure, systemic vascular resistance (SVR) and tachycardia (sympathetic stimulation).

Sevoflurane (Figure 9.1(b))

Sevoflurane has a low blood/gas solubility coefficient (0.69) and is non-irritant; it is therefore useful for inhalational induction. It causes bradycardia, blood pressure and SVR but cardiac output is maintained.

Desflurane (Figure 9.1(c))

Desflurane is a respiratory irritant and cannot be used for induction of anaesthesia. It increases salivary and respiratory secretions; CVS effects are similar to isoflurane. Recovery is rapid due to a low blood/gas solubility coefficient (0.42). Its boiling point is close to room temperature, and therefore it is used in a special vaporizer, which heats and pressurizes the desflurane so that the amount of vapour available is independent of ambient temperature.

Halothane (Figure 9.1(d))

Halothane is a halogenated hydrocarbon, still used in some parts of the world but mainly replaced due to side effects, including myocardial depression, myocardial sensitization to catecholamines and hepatitis. The cause of hepatitis is not fully understood but is thought to be related to repeated exposure; it has a very low incidence, presentation ranging from mild derangement of liver function tests to fulminant hepatic failure.

All volatile anaesthetics can trigger MH (see Chapter 23).

Nitrous oxide

This is a colourless, non-flammable gas at room temperature with a low molecular weight (44); it is relatively non-polar and highly lipid soluble. Its low potency means it cannot be used as a sole anaesthetic agent. Rapid equilibration between brain and inhaled concentration is due to its low blood/gas solubility coefficient. It is much more soluble than nitrogen, diffusing into air-filled spaces quicker than nitrogen can diffuse out. Situations where this might be a problem include:

- endotracheal cuff expansion (potential for mucosal damage);
- bowel expansion;
- a simple pneumothorax might become a tension pneumothorax;
- air emboli (a small insignificant embolus might enlarge);
- tympanic membrane bulging (middle ear surgery).

Its main side effect is PONV. It also inhibits methionine synthetase, involved in vitamin B_{12} production – megaloblastic anaemia is a theoretical complication with prolonged use.

The mechanism of action is not fully understood but it has been shown to be an NMDA antagonist as well as having action on opioid receptors.

Diffusional hypoxia – at the end of an anaesthetic, when nitrous oxide is stopped, it diffuses out of the tissues and blood into the alveolar gas, down its concentration gradient, at a rate greater than nitrogen uptake. This will dilute the oxygen present in the alveoli, resulting in the potential for hypoxia because the capillary blood is now exposed to a low oxygen concentration. This is avoided by giving the patient 100% O_2 at emergence.

Entonox is an equal mixture of N_2O and O_2. It is stored as a gas, as oxygen lowers the mixture's critical temperature to $-7°C$. If cylinders of Entonox are exposed to such temperatures, they should not be used until they have been exposed to a temperature of $>5°C$ for >24 hours. The concern is that liquid N_2O will be present, with an oxygen-rich mixture given initially (gaseous O_2) followed by a hypoxic N_2O-rich mixture as the O_2 becomes depleted.

Oxygen

This is manufactured by fractional distillation of air and is available via pipeline (at 4 bar) and cylinders (at 137 bar). It is stored in a vacuum insulated evaporator (VIE), separate from other hospital buildings. A VIE stores liquid O_2 with gaseous oxygen above. It provides O_2 throughout the hospital, with extra liquid O_2 being heated to the gas phase when demand is high. A safety valve allows venting of O_2 to the atmosphere when low demand causes a pressure build up.

Xenon

Xenon is a noble gas and exhibits many properties of an ideal anaesthetic agent (Table 9.3): colourless, odourless, non-flammable, stable in storage, low oil/gas and blood/gas coefficients, cardiovascularly stable, excreted unmetabolized, non-toxic, MH safe and not a greenhouse gas. However, it is very expensive (2000 times as expensive as N_2O).

10 General anaesthesia – intravenous anaesthetics

Figure 10.1 GABA_A receptor

- About 30% of all inhibitory synapses within the CNS are mediated by GABA_A receptors
- These consist of 5 subunits around a central ion channel; 2 alpha, 2 beta and 1 gamma. There are subtypes of the subunits and approximately 30 isoform combinations exist
- GABA binds to the interface between the alpha and beta subunits, which causes a conformational change in subunit-linked transmembrane proteins (transmembrane domain), causing the ion channel to open
- Anions (mainly chloride) enter the cell down their electrochemical gradient, causing hyperpolarization, and therefore inhibition, of the neurone. Volatile and intravenous anaesthetics are believed to act at the GABA_A receptor complex – lower doses via the alpha subunits; higher concentrations directly on the chloride channel itself
- There are site-specific actions of anaesthetic drugs, e.g. in mice studies, the alpha 1 subunit is responsible for amnesia and sedation, the alpha 2 subunit for anxiolysis
- Other sites for general anaesthetic action include an inhibitory action at the NMDA receptor, as well as at sodium and potassium channels

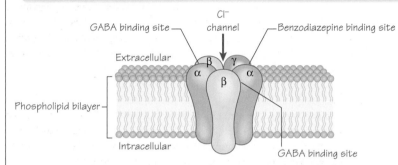

Events occurring during increased GABA receptor activity

1. GABA or anaesthetic bindings to receptor subunits
2. Conformational change of receptor
3. Chloride influx and hyperpolarization

Figure 10.2 Intravenous anaesthetics

Thiopentone

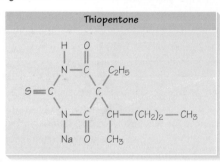

Propofol

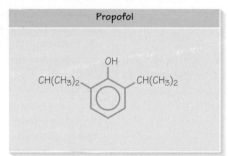

Etomidate

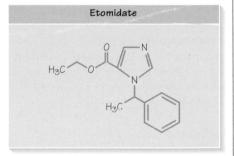

Ketamine

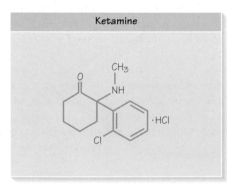

Midazolam

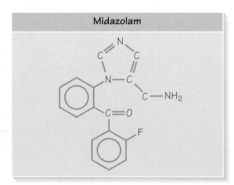

Midazolam is water soluble with an open ring structure. When exposed to physiological pH, the ring structure closes and it becomes highly lipophilic

---

The uses of intravenous anaesthetics are: induction and maintenance of anaesthesia, sedation (e.g. ITU) and operations under local anaesthesia.

Propofol (2,6-diisopropylphenol)

This is the commonest induction agent in current practice, and is most frequently used as a pre-prepared 1% (10 mg/mL) emulsion; it is highly lipid soluble.

It produces a smooth, rapid loss of consciousness after intravenous injection, with a relatively fast clinical recovery after either an induction dose or infusion, due to a short distribution half-life (1–2 min). It can cause discomfort on injection, alleviated by the addition of lidocaine.

The mechanism of action is unclear but it is thought to be an agonist at GABA receptors. Systemic effects include:

Anaesthesia at a Glance, First Edition. Julian Stone and William Fawcett.

CNS Dose-dependent sedation and hypnosis occur, with reduced cerebral blood flow, intracranial pressure and cerebral metabolic requirement for oxygen ($CMRO_2$). Its amnesic effect is less than barbiturates or benzodiazepines. Excitatory effects (e.g. involuntary movements) can occur but less commonly than with etomidate or thiopental. Anticonvulsant properties are exhibited although there are reports of grand mal seizures following its use. Hallucinations and sexual fantasies can occur.

CVS There is a marked fall in blood pressure due to direct myocardial depression, a reduction in systemic vascular resistance and a direct effect on vascular smooth muscle tone. This effect is more pronounced than with other agents.

RS Respiratory depression occurs, with a reduced response to hypercarbia and hypoxia. This reduced responsiveness is to a similar degree to that with barbiturates and volatile agents. Apnoea is common, especially if opiates or depressant premedications are used.

It produces laryngeal and pharyngeal muscle relaxation, allowing insertion of a laryngeal mask airway. It produces better laryngeal muscle relaxation than barbiturates and can be used with a short-acting opiate (with no muscle relaxant) to intubate the trachea.

Other advantages are:
• safe in malignant hyperthermia (MH) patients;
• safe in porphyria;
• antiemetic properties (valuable in patients with PONV risk);
• use in day case surgery where minimal postoperative hangover (e.g. drowsiness and ataxia) is desirable;
• situations where volatile anaesthetics cannot be used (e.g. MH, transfer of sedated patients, airway surgery when periods of apnoeic oxygenation are employed).

Total intravenous anaesthesia (TIVA) most commonly uses a propofol infusion to maintain anaesthesia. Specialized infusion pumps are used, delivering propofol at a rate that can give a predetermined plasma concentration (target controlled infusion).

Propofol emulsion also contains egg phosphatide and so care must be taken with patients who have an egg allergy.

Thiopental

This is a thiobarbiturate. It produces rapid loss of consciousness after intravenous injection; initial drug distribution is to vessel-rich tissues (e.g. brain). Return of consciousness then occurs with redistribution to lean tissue (e.g. muscle) and a further slower redistribution to vessel-poor tissues (e.g. fat). In plasma it is 85% protein bound.

Metabolism and elimination is hepatic. At high plasma concentrations (higher than those met in clinical anaesthesia) it saturates the P450 cytochromes, resulting in zero-order kinetics. Due to its slow metabolism it is not suitable for maintenance of anaesthesia.

CNS Thiopental reduces $CMRO_2$, cerebral blood flow and intracranial pressure. It has potent anticonvulsant properties.

CVS It causes venodilatation and reduced preload. SVR and arterial blood pressure are well maintained. It causes tachycardia and increases myocardial oxygen consumption. This is normally adequately compensated for by an increase in coronary blood flow but can lead to ischemia in patients with coronary stenosis or in hypovolaemia.

RS Dose-dependent respiratory depression and apnoea occurs. The response to both hypoxia and hypercapnia are reduced. Laryngeal and tracheal reflexes are suppressed to a lesser degree than with propofol. Anaesthesia is caused by its potentiation of GABA receptors.

Adverse effects include dose-dependent histamine release. It causes pain and inflammation if injected subcutaneously (e.g. into a cannula that has 'tissued'). Inadvertent intra-arterial injection produces acute pain and arteritis. Thiopental is less suitable for day case surgery due to its hangover effect. It is contraindicated in porphyria.

Benzodiazepines (e.g. midazolam)
• The effects of benzodiazepines are: anxiolytic, anticonvulsant, amnesic, sedative and hypnotic.
• Onset is rapid but slower than propofol or thiopental.
• They bind to the $GABA_A$ receptor complex and increase chloride ion influx, resulting in neuronal hyperpolarization (Figure 10.1).
• They have relative CVS stability.
• They cause mild respiratory depression but this can be marked and lead to apnoea in the elderly, with associated respiratory disease or with concurrent use of other respiratory depressant drugs (e.g. opiates).
• Flumazenil is a specific competitive antagonist. It has a short half-life (1 hour) and so care must be taken with reappearance of sedation after it is given to reverse the effect of longer-acting benzodiazepines (e.g. diazepam).

Ketamine
Ketamine is a phencyclidine derivative (Figure 10.2), which acts as an NMDA receptor antagonist and is highly lipid soluble with a rapid onset of action. It causes 'dissociative anaesthesia' with loss of consciousness and profound analgesia and as a result has abuse potential.

CVS HR and BP increase, whilst cardiac output (CO) is maintained. This is due to direct myocardial stimulation and a central sympathetic effect.

RS There is minimal respiratory depression, bronchodilatation occurs, and laryngeal/pharyngeal reflexes are preserved.

CNS The effects are analgesia, increased cerebral blood flow and intracranial pressure.

Other side effects These include PONV, increased salivation and increased uterine tone.

Ketamine's CVS stability makes it a useful drug for anaesthetic induction in shocked patients. The preservation of airway reflexes and less respiratory depression makes it suitable for procedures such as radiological interventions, radiotherapy, burns and dressing changes, especially with its associated analgesic effect. It has an opioid-sparing effect and can be used in PCAs.

It is avoided in ischaemic heart disease, hypertension, pre-eclampsia and raised intracranial pressure.

Etomidate
Etomidate is a carboxylated imidazole. It is short acting and potent, with CVS and RS stability, so is useful in elderly and shocked patients.

The disadvantages include:
• PONV;
• excitatory phenomena (e.g. involuntary limb twitches);
• myoclonus;
• inhibition of corticosteroid synthesis (11-β-hydroylase and 17-α-hydroylase), resulting in a reduction in the steroid stress response.

11 Local anaesthetics

Figure 11.1 General chemical structure of local anaesthetics showing aromatic ring, amine and the ester or amide linkage between them

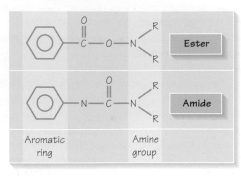

Table 11.1 Characteristics of local anaesthetics

Local anaesthetic	pKa	Maximum dose (mg/kg)	% protein binding
Ester			
Amethocaine	8.5	1.5	76
Cocaine	8.7	3	–
Procaine	8.9	12	6
Amide			
Bupivacaine	8.1	2	96
Lidocaine	7.9	3–7	64
Prilocaine	7.9	5–8	55
Ropivacaine	8.1	3.5	94

Figure 11.2 Lipid bilayer with a sodium channel, the site of action of local anaesthetics. Unionized LAs are able to cross the cell membrane but ionized LAs cannot

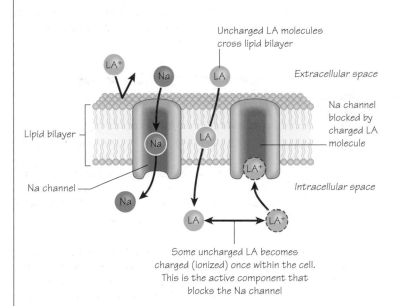

Figure 11.3 Rate of LA absorption

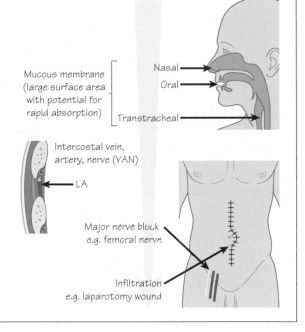

Local anaesthetics (LAs) are weak bases. They are divided into two groups, depending on the linkage between an aromatic ring and an amine group (Table 11.1). This linkage is either an amide or an ester (Figure 11.1).

Esters (e.g. cocaine, procaine, amethocaine) Allergic reactions are common. Metabolized by plasma and liver cholinesterase.

Amides (e.g. bupivacaine, lidocaine, ropivacaine) Allergic reactions are rare. Metabolized by the liver.

Uses

The uses of LAs include:
• local infiltration, e.g. laceration suturing, postoperatively to surgical wounds;
• topical to mucous membrane, e.g. cornea, nose, oropharynx;
• spinal cord – epidural and spinal;
• minor nerve blockade, e.g. radial nerve;
• major nerve trunk blockade, e.g. brachial plexus block;
• intravenous regional anaesthesia – Bier's block with prilocaine or lidocaine;
• cardiac tachydysrhythmias, e.g. lidocaine for ventricular tachycardia (VT);
• topical to skin – eutectic mixture of local anaesthetics (EMLA), amethocaine;
• reducing discomfort of propofol injection, e.g. by adding 10 mg lidocaine.

Mechanism of action

LAs act by reversible inhibition of action potential transmission in all excitable tissues. They block sodium channels of nerve cell mem-

Anaesthesia at a Glance, First Edition. Julian Stone and William Fawcett.

branes and prevent sodium influx and action potential propagation and hence nerve conduction (Figure 11.2). Only the non-polar (lipophilic) form of the drug can cross the cell membrane and, once intracellular, the polar component becomes the active drug, which blocks the channel. The higher the frequency of sodium channel opening, the more susceptible is the nerve to blockade – hence sensory nerve fibres are blocked before motor nerves.

Speed of onset of action

This is related to the amount of drug in the unionized form that can cross the cell membrane. This depends on its pKa (pH at which 50% of the drug is in the ionized form); for example lidocaine (pKa 7.9) has a quicker speed of onset than bupivacaine (pKa 8.1) because more lidocaine is unionized at physiological pH and hence can cross the cell membrane.

Additives effect the speed of onset; for example bicarbonate raises extracellular pH and thus increases the unionized fraction of the drug, which can then cross the cell membrane.

Duration of action

Protein-bound LAs have a longer duration of action. Ester LAs may have a prolonged duration of action when plasma cholinesterase is reduced, for example in pregnancy, liver disease or when the enzyme is atypical or absent (e.g. pseudocholinesterase deficiency).

The duration of action may be prolonged by the addition of vaso-constrictors to the LA to reduce systemic absorption (e.g. epinephrine or felypressin). These aim to keep the LA concentrated at its site of administration to prolong its action, reduce toxicity and possibly enhance block quality. LA with a vasoconstrictor should never be used in areas with terminal arterial blood supplies where necrosis can result (e.g. digits or penis). When some LAs are used with a vasoconstrictor, their maximum safe dose increases (e.g. lidocaine on its own = 3 mg/kg, with epinephrine = 7 mg/kg). Others (e.g. bupivacaine) remain unchanged when epinephrine is used.

Hyperbaric solutions of LA (e.g. by the addition of dextrose) effect the spread of LA when injected into the CSF. Dextrose is denser than CSF and when combined in solution causes the LA to sink to the most dependent part, that is to the left or right if the patient is lying on their side or to the caudal area if sitting upright.

LA potency is related to lipid solubility.

Toxicity

This occurs as a result of membrane stabilization of other excitable tissues (e.g. CNS, heart). Toxicity can be due to an excessive dose of drug being given or due to a smaller dose being given inadvertently via the wrong route (e.g. intravenously) (Figure 11.3).

Features include circumoral tingling, feeling of impending doom, dysrhythmias, CVS collapse, loss of consciousness, convulsions and cardiac arrest.

Treatment is supportive, including airway maintenance/endotracheal intubation if needed, intravenous fluids and vasopressors (e.g. epinephrine), and control of seizures with, for example, benzodiazepines, thiopental or propofol. If cardiac arrest has occurred then CPR is performed.

Intravenous lipid emulsion Intralipid (Baxter, Newbury, Berkshire) 20% 1.5 mL/kg is now recommended for LA toxicity/cardiovascular collapse. Recovery can take more than an hour so CPR may be prolonged.

The rate of systemic absorption depends on the site of administration: mucous membranes >intercostals >major nerve block >infiltration (see Figure 11.3).

Bupivacaine consists of both levo- and dextroisomers. The former is associated with less serious CNS and CVS toxicity, and levobupivacaine is increasingly being used in place of racemic bupivacaine.

Other side effects

Allergy is common with the esters, especially with procaine (causative metabolite is *para*-aminobenzoic acid) but very rare with amides. It is more likely to be related to additives such as vasoconstrictors or preservatives.

Prilocaine metabolism produces toludine, which reduces Hb to metHb. Excess prilocine can therefore cause methaemoglobinaemia. It is treated with methylene blue.

Eutectic mixture of local anaesthetics (EMLA) and intravenous regional anaesthesia (IVRA)

EMLA This is an emulsion of equal amounts of the base forms of prilocaine and lidocaine. (*Eutektos* (Greek) means easily melted.) Each drug lowers the melting point of the other. It provides surface anaesthesia when applied to skin and left for an adequate time to work (>45 min). It is useful for paediatrics and dressing changes. Amethocaine gel is also available and has a quicker onset than EMLA. Other forms of LA are poorly absorbed through intact skin.

Bier's block (IVRA) A BP cuff is applied to the upper arm after placement of a cannula in the hand. After exsanguination of the limb by either elevation or the use of a compression bandage, the BP cuff is inflated to 100 mmHg above systolic BP. Prilocaine is the preferred drug and is injected i.v. It is unable to spread beyond the cuff and thus acts within the confined area. This provides good analgesia for distal limb procedures (e.g. fracture manipulation or carpel tunnel decompression). The cuff is let down after at least 20 min to allow the LA to spread into the adjacent tissues in order to prevent toxic plasma levels of LA following systemic absorption. A second cannula must always be sited in the other arm for emergency use.

12 Neuromuscular blocking drugs

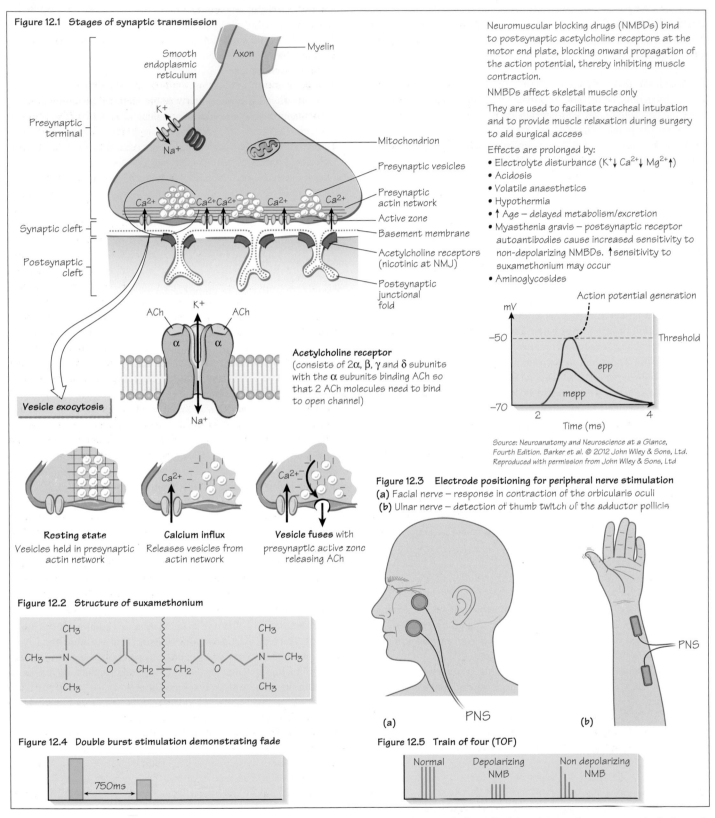

Figure 12.1 Stages of synaptic transmission

Smooth endoplasmic reticulum
Axon
Myelin
K+
Na+
Presynaptic terminal
Mitochondrion
Presynaptic vesicles
Presynaptic actin network
Active zone
Ca^{2+} Ca^{2+} Ca^{2+} Ca^{2+} Ca^{2+}
Synaptic cleft
Basement membrane
Acetylcholine receptors (nicotinic at NMJ)
Postsynaptic cleft
Postsynaptic junctional fold

Vesicle exocytosis

ACh K+ ACh
α α
Na+

Acetylcholine receptor
(consists of 2α, β, γ and δ subunits with the α subunits binding ACh so that 2 ACh molecules need to bind to open channel)

Resting state
Vesicles held in presynaptic actin network

Calcium influx
Releases vesicles from actin network
Ca^{2+}

Vesicle fuses with presynaptic active zone releasing ACh
Ca^{2+}

Neuromuscular blocking drugs (NMBDs) bind to postsynaptic acetylcholine receptors at the motor end plate, blocking onward propagation of the action potential, thereby inhibiting muscle contraction.

NMBDs affect skeletal muscle only

They are used to facilitate tracheal intubation and to provide muscle relaxation during surgery to aid surgical access

Effects are prolonged by:
- Electrolyte disturbance ($K^+\downarrow$ $Ca^{2+}\downarrow$ $Mg^{2+}\uparrow$)
- Acidosis
- Volatile anaesthetics
- Hypothermia
- $\uparrow$ Age – delayed metabolism/excretion
- Myasthenia gravis – postsynaptic receptor autoantibodies cause increased sensitivity to non-depolarizing NMBDs. $\uparrow$sensitivity to suxamethonium may occur
- Aminoglycosides

Action potential generation
mV
−50 Threshold
epp
mepp
−70
2 Time (ms) 4

Source: Neuroanatomy and Neuroscience at a Glance, Fourth Edition. Barker et al. © 2012 John Wiley & Sons, Ltd. Reproduced with permission from John Wiley & Sons, Ltd

Figure 12.3 Electrode positioning for peripheral nerve stimulation
(a) Facial nerve – response in contraction of the orbicularis oculi
(b) Ulnar nerve – detection of thumb twitch of the adductor pollicis

PNS
(a)
PNS
(b)

Figure 12.2 Structure of suxamethonium

CH_3 CH_3
CH_3—N—CH_2—O—CH_2 CH_2—O—N—CH_3
CH_3 CH_3

Figure 12.4 Double burst stimulation demonstrating fade
750ms

Figure 12.5 Train of four (TOF)
Normal Depolarizing NMB Non depolarizing NMB

Acetylcholine (ACh) is the neurotransmitter at skeletal muscle synaptic junctions. It is synthesized from choline and acetyl coenzyme A by acetylcholinetransferase and stored in presynaptic vesicles. An action potential causes influx of calcium ions at the nerve terminal, the vesicles then move into the active zone and fuse with the axonal membrane. The active zones lie opposite the postsynaptic membrane ACh

Anaesthesia at a Glance, First Edition. Julian Stone and William Fawcett.

receptors. An action potential causes 200–300 vesicles to release their quanta of ACh into the space between the nerve terminal and the muscle membrane (the junctional cleft) (Figure 12.1).

The ACh binds to the two alpha subunits of the ACh receptor, causing its ionophore to briefly open and allowing ion flux (mainly Na^+ influx followed by K^+ efflux). Spread of the action potential causes mobilization of Ca^{2+} from the sarcoplasmic reticulum and subsequent muscle contraction.

ACh is metabolized by acetylcholinesterase, present in the junctional cleft (60 nm wide) and postsynaptic membrane junctional folds. The choline produced by ACh breakdown is taken up for reuse.

Depolarizing neuromuscular blocking drugs (NMBDs) – suxamethonium

Suxamethonium consists of two ACh molecules connected by their acetyl groups (Figure 12.2). It binds to the postsynaptic ACh receptor, causing depolarization. In order for the ionophore to be reset for a further depolarization, ACh is metabolized in the cleft by acetylcholinesterase. However, suxamethonium is not metabolized by acetylcholinesterase and so produces initial fasciculation followed by a block, as no further action potential can be propagated whilst the suxamethonium is still bound to the receptor. It is subsequently metabolized by plasma cholinesterase.

It has the fastest onset (60 s) and shortest duration (approximately 10 min) of all NMBDs. Its main use is in endotracheal intubation when rapid intubating conditions are required. Its effect is antagonized by non-depolarizing NMBDs and potentiated by anticholinesterase inhibitors. Dual block may occur if excessive or repeated doses are given, resulting in features of a non-depolarizing block replacing those of a depolarizing block.

Suxamethonium has many side effects:
- MH (see Chapter 23);
- Suxamethonium apnoea – less plasma cholinesterase results in prolongation of effect due to inherited or acquired causes (e.g. liver disease, starvation, malignancy, cardiac failure, renal failure). The plasma cholinesterase gene inheritance is autosomal; abnormalities are more common in Asian and Middle Eastern patients. Its action may be prolonged by several minutes to hours. Management is supportive, especially to avoid awareness.
- anaphylaxis;
- hyperkalaemia – care must be taken in patients with renal failure, burns, muscular dystrophies and paraplegia (extrajunctional ACh receptor proliferation);
- histamine release;
- bradycardia ;
- dual block;
- raised intraocular pressure;
- myalgia.

Non-depolarizing neuromuscular blocking drugs

Non-depolarizing NMBDs have a slower onset than suxamethonium and provide reversible competitive antagonism at the neuromuscular junction with ACh. Blockade starts when 70–80% of receptors at the junction are blocked, and is complete with 90% blockade. They are highly ionized, poorly lipid soluble and protein bound at physiological pH. Muscle function returns as the drug diffuses out into the plasma; none is metabolized within the junction.

There are two main types of non-depolarizing NMBDs:

- Benzylisoquinoliniums, e.g.
  - **atracurium:** metabolized spontaneously in plasma by Hofmann degradation and causes histamine release;
  - **cisatracurium:** an atracurium isomer, causing less histamine release;
  - **mivacurium:** short acting and metabolized by plasma cholinesterase.
- Aminosteroids, e.g.
  - **pancuronium:** long acting, cardiovascular stability;
  - **vecuronium:** cardiovascularly stable, minimal histamine release;
  - **rocuronium:** fastest onset of non-depolarizing NMBDs. Minimal histamine release and is cardiovascularly stable, although it is vagolytic at higher doses, producing tachycardia. It has a long duration of action (40 min).

All non-depolarizing NMBDs have at least one ammonium group, the active part, which binds to postsynaptic ACh receptor alpha subunits.

Reversal of residual NMBDs is almost always required at the end of surgery. Residual weakness is very unpleasant for patients and puts them at risk postoperatively of inadequate breathing and airway protection. Anticholinesterases bind with the esteratic site of the acetylcholinesterase, increasing ACh concentrations. The only commonly used anticholinesterase in anaesthesia is neostigmine. However, it not only causes increased levels of ACh at the nicotinic receptors (at the neuromuscular junction) but also at muscarinic ACh receptors, causing bradycardia, bronchospasm, increased bronchial secretions, sweating, salivation and gastrointestinal upset. Therefore neostigmine is always administered with an antimuscarinic drug (e.g. glycopyrronium or atropine).

Sugammadex (a cyclodextrin) binds irreversibly to rocuronium and vecuronium, rendering them inactive. It has a role in failed intubation/ventilation scenarios by reversing muscle relaxation when rapid resumption of airway reflexes and respiratory function is required.

Monitoring of muscle paralysis

Neuromuscular blockade monitoring For this a nerve stimulator applies a current to a peripheral nerve and the motor response is observed. Common sites include facial nerve (facial twitch) and ulnar nerve (thumb abduction) (Figure 12.3a,b). A current of uniform amplitude (20–60 mA) is applied; a supramaximal stimulus ensures depolarization of all nerves within a nerve fibre. The current is of short duration (0.1–0.2 ms). Assessment is most commonly by tactile and visual assessment of elicited muscle twitches – the easiest but least accurate technique. Other methods include electromyography, acceleromyography and mechanomyography (using a strain gauge).

Fade This is a progressive diminution of muscle twitch when four stimuli (at 2 Hz) are applied (Figure 12.4). The ratio of the fourth to first twitch amplitude is called the train of four ratio (TOF). As the degree of block increases, the twitches disappear from the fourth to first, with recovery in the opposite order (Figure 12.5).

Facilitation This is used to assess profound block. After a tetanic stimulus (e.g. 5 s at 50 Hz) there is enhanced response to single twitches, thought to be due to presynaptic mobilization of ACh. The number of single twitches elicited is the post-tetanic count, which can be used to determine recovery time and can be used when TOF is undetectable.

Double burst stimulation This is two 50-Hz stimuli separated by 750 ms. It is thought to be a more accurate visual assessment *of fade* than TOF.

13 Acute pain

Figure 13.1 Classic pain pathway

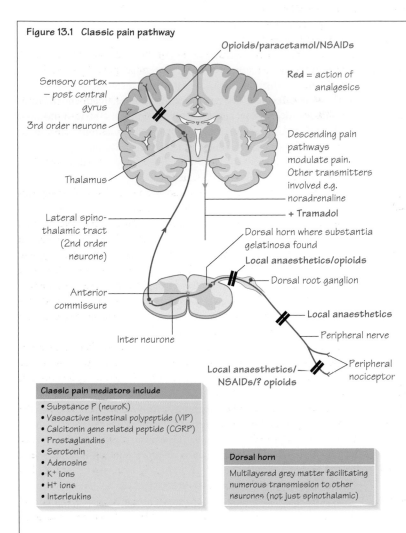

Opioids/paracetamol/NSAIDs

Red = action of analgesics

- Sensory cortex – post central gyrus
- 3rd order neurone
- Thalamus
- Lateral spino-thalamic tract (2nd order neurone)
- Anterior commissure
- Inter neurone

Descending pain pathways modulate pain. Other transmitters involved e.g. noradrenaline
+ Tramadol

- Dorsal horn where substantia gelatinosa found
- Local anaesthetics/opioids
- Dorsal root ganglion
- Local anaesthetics
- Peripheral nerve
- Local anaesthetics/NSAIDs/? opioids
- Peripheral nociceptor

Classic pain mediators include

- Substance P (neuroK)
- Vasoactive intestinal polypeptide (VIP)
- Calcitonin gene related peptide (CGRP)
- Prostaglandins
- Serotonin
- Adenosine
- K^+ ions
- H^+ ions
- Interleukins

Dorsal horn

Multilayered grey matter facilitating numerous transmission to other neurones (not just spinothalamic)

Figure 13.2 Gate theory of pain

Pain fibres (green) cause inhibition of the interneuron (**i**) and facilitate onward transmission by the transmission cell (**t**) to the CNS. Large fibre afferents (yellow) stimulate the interneuron, itself causing inhibition to the input of the t cell. Descending inhibition will also reduce transmission

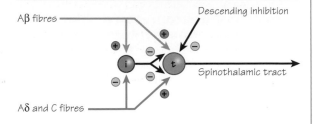

Aβ fibres
Descending inhibition
Spinothalamic tract
Aδ and C fibres

Figure 13. 3 WHO pain relief ladder

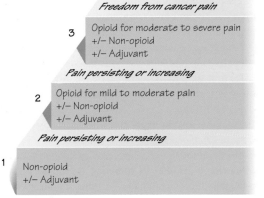

Freedom from cancer pain

3 Opioid for moderate to severe pain
+/– Non-opioid
+/– Adjuvant

Pain persisting or increasing

2 Opioid for mild to moderate pain
+/– Non-opioid
+/– Adjuvant

Pain persisting or increasing

1 Non-opioid
+/– Adjuvant

Reprinted with kind permission from WHO

Table 13.1 Transmitters involved in pain pathways

Type	Example
Opioid peptides	Endorphins, encephalins
Amines	Noradrenaline and 5-HT
Excitatory amino acids	Glutamate
Inhibitory amino acids	GABA, Glycine
Other peptides	Substance P

Table 13.3 Effects of drugs in the epidural space

Local anaesthetics	• Sensory block – pain relief, urinary retention • Motor block – paralysis, urinary retention • Sympathetic block – hypotension
Opioids	• Respiratory depression • Urinary retention • Itching

Table 13.2 Typical patient-controlled analgesia (PCA) settings

Drug	Morphine
Bolus	1 mg
Lockout time	5 minutes
4-Hour limit	20 mg
Background	Nil

Table 13.4 Risk and benefits of epidural infusions

Benefits	Risks

• Superlative pain relief
• Opioid sparing
• Quicker return of GI function
• Reduction in:
  • Pulmonary thromboembolism
  • Blood loss and transfusion
  • Some respiratory complications
  • Stress response
	• Hypotension and its risks (MI, renal failure, CVA and side effects of excess fluid administration)
	• Poor mobility
	• Permanent neurological damage

Anaesthesia at a Glance, First Edition. Julian Stone and William Fawcett.

Acute pain requires immediate intervention. Not only is it a basic humanitarian duty to treat pain, but untreated pain also has a number of adverse sequelae:

• Patients may not be able to mobilize adequately, predisposing to increased risk of DVT and inability to cooperate with physiotherapy.

• For abdominal and thoracic surgery unresolved pain may cause the patient to breathe at low lung volumes. This, in combination with decreased ability to cough, results in basal airway closure and retention of pulmonary secretions, leading into a spiral of hypoxia, lung collapse and predisposition to bacterial infection (pneumonia).

• Severe pain may cause a marked sympathetic response (tachycardia and hypertension), which are undesirable especially in patients with heart disease (e.g. angina).

Pain following surgery is usually relatively short lived and even following the most painful operations (thoracic and upper abdominal) is significantly reduced in intensity by 48–72 hours. Peripheral surgery may only necessitate pain control for 24 hours or so. Patients need to have their pain control discussed in advance so they know how it will be managed. Although much of acute pain is postoperative, there are many other causes: preoperative surgical (renal colic, peritonitis), medical (acute MI) and trauma (rib fractures).

The pain pathway (Figure 13.1) is fundamental to appreciating the mechanism of action of different analgesics and understanding multimodal analgesia. Pain from pain nerve endings (nociceptors) produces a signal that is carried to the dorsal horn of the spinal cord. The are two nerve pathways: sharp pain is transmitted by myelinated Aδ fibres and duller-onset pain is transmitted by unmyelinated C fibres.

There are numerous transmitters involved in pain transmission (Table 13.1). At the spinal cord level the impulses are transmitted to the thalamus by the spinothalamic tract. From there, neurons project to the somatosensory area in the postcentral gyrus where the pain is perceived.

At various stages in the pain pathway the process can be modulated or changed, thus similar injuries can produce vastly different perceptions. Modulation includes the following mechanisms:

• According to the Gate Theory (Figure 13.2), pain fibres 'open the gate', facilitating onward transmission. However, simultaneous input by Aβ fibres causes an inhibitory interneuron to stop this process 'closing the gate', explaining the reduction in pain intensity from rubbing the area or a Transcutaneous Electrical Nerve Stimulation (TENS) machine.

• Spinal cord activity can also be modulated via more complex mechanisms, e.g. from descending pathways from the brain stem.

Pain management

In spite of the complexities in physiology, the principles of managing acute pain are relatively straightforward.

1 The **WHO ladder** describes management of cancer pain (Figure 13.3) but the principles are similar for acute pain. The patient initially receives simple (non-opioid) analgesics (NSAIDs and paracetamol), if necessary moving to moderate opioids (codeine or tramadol) and finally strong opioids (e.g. morphine).

2 **Multimodal analgesia** (also discussed in Chapter 34, Table 13.2). The use of drugs with different mechanisms of action, often with synergistic effects, results in a reduction in necessary dose and adverse effects, particularly the opioids ('opioid sparing'). Commonly used drugs in acute pain include:

(a) opioids

(b) NSAIDs

(c) paracetamol

(d) local anaesthetics.

For many postoperative patients all of these drugs may be used. Newer/experimental approaches are ketamine plus PCA and oral pregabalin.

3 The **side effects of the analgesics** may need treatment. Opioids (respiratory depression, nausea and vomiting, constipation) and NSAIDs (renal impairment, bleeding and gastrointestinal perforation) account for many side effects.

4 **Prescribing regular analgesics** for 48–72 hours ensures that drug levels and hence analgesia is optimized.

5 **Infusion devices** also provide a more constant level of analgesics drugs; two major devices in common use are:

(a) **Patient-controlled analgesia** (PCA). This device consists of a container of opioid (usually morphine) and a handset. The patient presses the handset to get a bolus of morphine intravenously. Typical settings are shown in Table 13.2. PCA provides blood levels of morphine and hence analgesia that are rapidly titrated to the patients' needs. Nurse-controlled analgesia (NCA), in which i.v. opioids are administered by a nurse, can be used for those unable to operate the handset themselves (typically children).

(b) **Epidural infusions**. Typically, both local anaesthetic (e.g. bupivacaine) and opioid (e.g. fentanyl) are used. The epidural can be inserted in the lumbar or thoracic region. The physiological effects, benefits and side effects are shown in Tables 13.3 and 13.4.

Other devices may be used to infuse local anaesthetics into the wound or around major nerves, e.g. brachial plexus.

6 **Nausea and vomiting**. Patients should be prescribed antiemetics and the use of a combination of various treatments is useful, e.g. phenothiazine (prochlorperazine) 5-HT$_3$ receptor antagonists (ondansetron), steroids (dexamethasone).

7 **Patient monitoring and pain scoring**. Safety is paramount and patients need to be observed and the effects of analgesia documented.

(a) **Monitoring**. In addition to the usual pulse, blood pressure and respiratory rate measurements, sedation should be monitored as it may reflect excess opioid administration. Nausea and vomiting should also be assessed. With epidurals, the height of the block must also be measured. Onset of severe weakness and back pain may indicate an epidural haematoma/abscess and requires urgent investigation (MRI). Many hospitals have a scoring system for sedation, nausea and vomiting and leg weakness.

(b) **Pain score**. The documentation of pain scores, either on a numerical scale or a visual analogue scale, both at pain and at rest, should be undertaken. High pain scores require intervention, and the effect of this intervention can also be assessed.

Patients will need to be in an environment where appropriate observations and intervention can be performed. The location will depend on the patient and the type of pain control, e.g. elderly patients with thoracic epidural infusion may require level 1 care (high dependency).

14 Postoperative nausea and vomiting

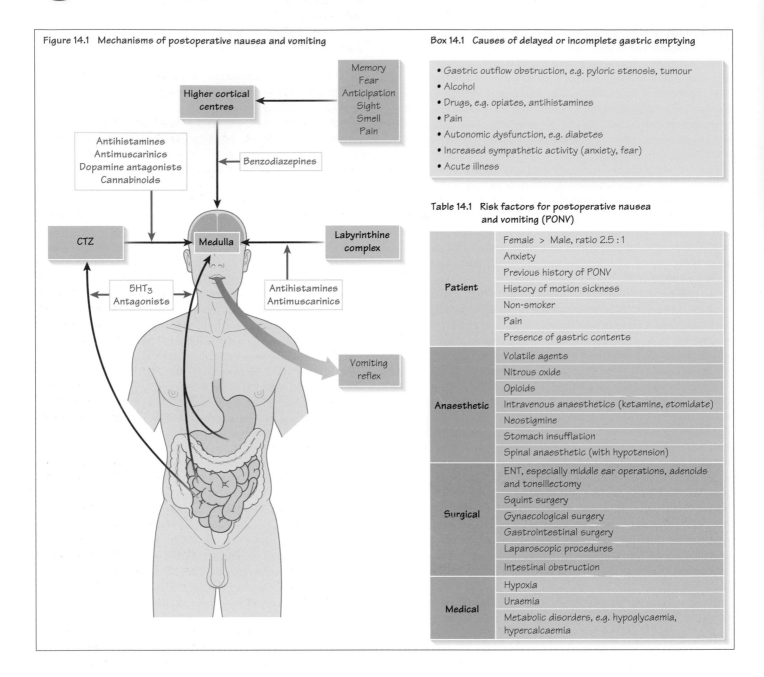

Figure 14.1 Mechanisms of postoperative nausea and vomiting

Box 14.1 Causes of delayed or incomplete gastric emptying

- Gastric outflow obstruction, e.g. pyloric stenosis, tumour
- Alcohol
- Drugs, e.g. opiates, antihistamines
- Pain
- Autonomic dysfunction, e.g. diabetes
- Increased sympathetic activity (anxiety, fear)
- Acute illness

Table 14.1 Risk factors for postoperative nausea and vomiting (PONV)

Patient	Female > Male, ratio 2.5 : 1
	Anxiety
	Previous history of PONV
	History of motion sickness
	Non-smoker
	Pain
	Presence of gastric contents
Anaesthetic	Volatile agents
	Nitrous oxide
	Opioids
	Intravenous anaesthetics (ketamine, etomidate)
	Neostigmine
	Stomach insufflation
	Spinal anaesthetic (with hypotension)
Surgical	ENT, especially middle ear operations, adenoids and tonsillectomy
	Squint surgery
	Gynaecological surgery
	Gastrointestinal surgery
	Laparoscopic procedures
	Intestinal obstruction
Medical	Hypoxia
	Uraemia
	Metabolic disorders, e.g. hypoglycaemia, hypercalcaemia

The overall incidence of postoperative nausea and vomiting (PONV) is approximately 30% but can be as high as 80%. It is not only unpleasant and distressing for the patient, but also has important medical consequences:
- aspiration of gastric contents (especially in the recovery period following an anaesthetic when protective airway reflexes might not have fully returned);
- dehydration and electrolyte disturbance;
- increased intraocular and intracranial pressure in susceptible patients;
- delayed hospital discharge, and the need for day surgery patients to be admitted overnight;
- it is unpleasant and can lead to increased anxiety for subsequent operations.

Mechanism

Afferent nerve fibres (mainly vagal) from the GI tract supply the chemoreceptor trigger zone (CTZ) which is situated in the area postrema in the caudal part of the floor of the 4th ventricle. There are both mechanoreceptors (detecting gut wall distension, e.g. in bowel obstruction) and chemoreceptors (detecting toxins etc.). Other afferents (e.g. higher cortical centres, vestibular apparatus) converge on the CTZ. The CTZ lies outside both the blood–brain barrier and the CSF–brain barrier, and so is able to detect stimulants to vomiting from both blood

Anaesthesia at a Glance, First Edition. Julian Stone and William Fawcett.

and CSF. The CTZ interacts with the vomiting centre (dorsolateral reticular formation of the medulla). Several receptors are involved: H_1, ACh (M_3), 5-HT_3 and dopamine (D_2) (Figure 14.1).

Treatment

Drug treatment

Most antiemetic drugs act on more than one receptor.

Antihistamines e.g. cyclizine. These act on H_1 central receptors (as opposed to H_2 gastric receptors). Cyclizine also has an anticholinergic action and causes tachycardia when given intravenously.

Anticholinergics e.g. atropine, hyoscine. These are non-polar so are able to cross the blood–brain barrier and act on muscarinic receptors in the vomiting centre and GI tract, reducing GI and salivary secretions and intestinal tone. They counteract motion and opiate-induced nausea and vomiting. Side effects include dry mouth, blurred vision and urinary retention.

Antidopaminergics

- Phenothiazines, e.g. prochlorperazine, act on D_2 receptors in the CTZ as well as having anticholinergic action (M3 receptors).
- Butyrophenones, e.g. droperidol, haloperidol, act by central D2 antagonism.
- Benzamides, e.g. metoclopramide, has D_2, H_1 and 5-HT_3 antagonism as well as increasing the speed of gastric emptying through the pylorus (prokinetic).

Extrapyramidal side effects (e.g. oculogyric crisis, dystonia, slurred speech) can occur with all dopamine antagonists. Treatment is with procyclidine.

Steroids e.g. dexamethasone. The mechanism of action is unclear (they also have multiple adverse side effects).

5-HT_3 antagonists e.g. ondansetron, granisetron. 5-HT_3 receptors are present in the area postrema as well as the GI tract. Dizziness, headache and constipation are their main side effects.

Benzodiazepines e.g. lorazepam, temazepam. They are used more commonly as prophylaxis in cancer chemotherapy, possibly acting as anxiolytics and reducing centrally mediated PONV pathways.

Cannabinoids e.g. nabilone. This is a synthetic analogue of the naturally occurring delta-9-tetrahydocannibol. CB1 receptors are present in the CNS, lung, liver and kidneys. Although not used routinely in PONV, they have a place in cancer chemotherapy nausea and vomiting.

Non-pharmacological treatment

Perioperative intravenous fluids Patients are often starved for many more hours than the minimum 2 hours for water and 6 hours for solids. Fluid resuscitation reduces PONV and the time to first oral intake.

Acupuncture Stimulation of the P6 acupuncture point preoperatively (2.5–5 cm proximal to the distal wrist crease between the flexor carpi radialis and palmaris longus tendons) reduces the incidence of PONV in adults but not children.

Hypnosis This may help in certain cases.

Ginger Results have been mixed. It is also used in motion sickness and pregnancy-related nausea and vomiting.

Vomiting is preceded by increased sympathetic (peripheral vasoconstriction, hyperventilation, sweating, papillary dilatation) and parasympathetic activity (salivation). Abdominal wall and diaphragmatic contraction causes expulsion of gastric contents, whilst breathing halts to prevent aspiration. Vomiting is an active process, whereas regurgitation occurs passively and is more likely to occur when conscious level is reduced, with a consequent increased risk of aspiration of vomit.

Management

At the preoperative assessment the anaesthetist will try to identify those patients who are at increased risk of PONV from the factors described above. Certain factors are unavoidable (most patient factors, the type of operation, etc.) but attention is paid to tailoring the anaesthetic to minimize the risk of PONV whilst at the same time ensuring that other factors (e.g. postoperative pain relief) are not compromised. Points to consider are:

- Delay surgery until the stomach empty, i.e. ensure that the patient has been starved of solids for 6 hours. In those patients who may have a full stomach after this time (see Box 14.1), give antacids and prokinetics (e.g. sodium citrate and metoclopramide) as appropriate to minimize the risk of regurgitation and PONV.
- Avoid prolonged bag mask ventilation.
- N_2O is thought to cause PONV by bowel and middle ear distension. Currently, it is being used less and should be avoided in patients who are thought to be at risk of PONV.
- Total intravenous anaesthesia (TIVA) is an anaesthetic technique in which the patient breathes oxygen-enriched air and anaesthesia is induced and maintained through intravenous agents only. This avoids both the use of N_2O and volatile anaesthetics. Propofol in this situation has the advantage of possessing antiemetic properties.
- Periods of hypotension should be avoided, especially if a spinal anaesthetic has been used.
- i.v. fluids are of benefit.
- Combination therapy with antiemetics acting on different sites and receptors (multimodal) is more effective than monotherapy, e.g. triple therapy using ondansetron, dexamethasone and droperidol.

15 Chronic pain

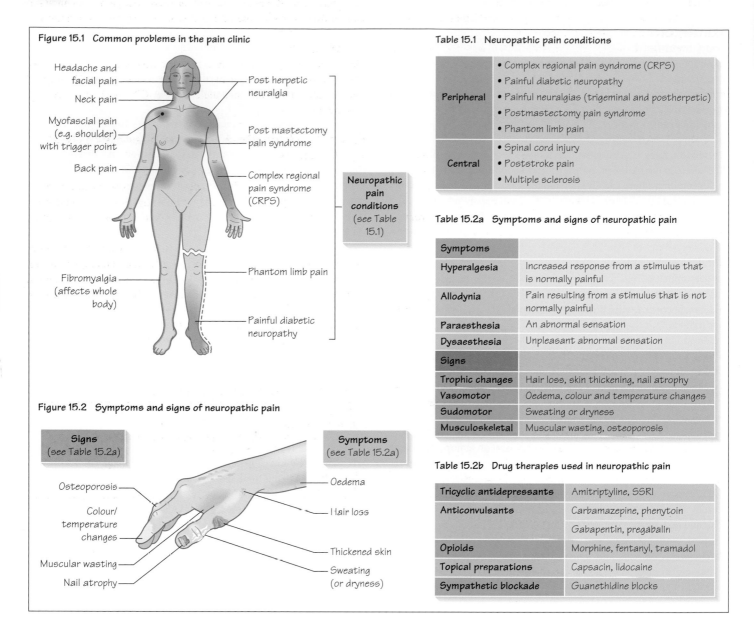

Figure 15.1 Common problems in the pain clinic

Headache and facial pain
Neck pain
Myofascial pain (e.g. shoulder) with trigger point
Back pain
Fibromyalgia (affects whole body)

Post herpetic neuralgia
Post mastectomy pain syndrome
Complex regional pain syndrome (CRPS)
Phantom limb pain
Painful diabetic neuropathy

Neuropathic pain conditions (see Table 15.1)

Table 15.1 Neuropathic pain conditions

Peripheral	• Complex regional pain syndrome (CRPS) • Painful diabetic neuropathy • Painful neuralgias (trigeminal and postherpetic) • Postmastectomy pain syndrome • Phantom limb pain
Central	• Spinal cord injury • Poststroke pain • Multiple sclerosis

Table 15.2a Symptoms and signs of neuropathic pain

Symptoms	
Hyperalgesia	Increased response from a stimulus that is normally painful
Allodynia	Pain resulting from a stimulus that is not normally painful
Paraesthesia	An abnormal sensation
Dysaesthesia	Unpleasant abnormal sensation
Signs	
Trophic changes	Hair loss, skin thickening, nail atrophy
Vasomotor	Oedema, colour and temperature changes
Sudomotor	Sweating or dryness
Musculoskeletal	Muscular wasting, osteoporosis

Figure 15.2 Symptoms and signs of neuropathic pain

Signs (see Table 15.2a)
Osteoporosis
Colour/temperature changes
Muscular wasting
Nail atrophy

Symptoms (see Table 15.2a)
Oedema
Hair loss
Thickened skin
Sweating (or dryness)

Table 15.2b Drug therapies used in neuropathic pain

Tricyclic antidepressants	Amitriptyline, SSRI
Anticonvulsants	Carbamazepine, phenytoin
	Gabapentin, pregabalin
Opioids	Morphine, fentanyl, tramadol
Topical preparations	Capsacin, lidocaine
Sympathetic blockade	Guanethidine blocks

Whilst acute pain is a self-limiting process and is usually a clinical entity for only a few days, chronic pain persists longer than the expected time of healing and becomes the illness itself rather than a symptom of it. In addition there are other changes, particularly psychological. Chronic pain represents a wide spectrum of disease entities (Figure 15.1).

The mechanisms and pathways involved in chronic pain may be different to acute (nociceptive) pain. An important feature of some chronic pain syndromes is neuropathic pain, which is caused by central nervous system dysfunction, and often results in pain long after any painful stimulus has disappeared. There are many proposed mechanisms, including spontaneous activity within the dorsal root ganglion (DRG) and sympathetic nerve sprouting into the DRG. Within the dorsal horn, changes may also occur due to a reduction in inhibitory influences. In addition, there may be rewiring so that Aβ fibres (carrying touch) are synapsing on pain fibres. This different mechanism of pain gives rise to different treatments; indeed, conventional analgesics for acute pain may be ineffective for neuropathic pain.

Neuropathic pain

Neuropathic pain may be classified as either peripheral or central (see Table 15.1).

There are a number of features of neuropathic pain, which are shown in Figure 15.2. A classical type of neuropathic pain, complex regional pain syndrome (CRPS), typifies this clinical condition. It may follow an injury (e.g. Colles fracture) or there may be no injury. There may also be varying degrees of sympathetic nervous system involvement. With sympathetically maintained pain a sympathetic blockade

Anaesthesia at a Glance, First Edition. Julian Stone and William Fawcett.

will alleviate pain, whereas with sympathetically independent pain sympathetic blockade will have little effect.

Treatments that are used in neuropathic pain are:
- **Drug therapies** (Figure 15.2c). Tricyclic antidepressants and/or anticonvulsants may be all that is required.
- **Physical interventions**. These include TENS, acupuncture, neuromodulation (spinal cord stimulation) and sympathetic nerve denervation.
- **Psychological therapies**. These include cognitive behavioural therapy (CBT).

Chronic back pain

This is pain lasting more than 3 months. It is a very common problem in the pain clinic and is a huge problem both for the NHS (in terms of resources used) and nationally (days lost through sick leave). Many cases will settle spontaneously. The vast majority of pain is categorized as musculoskeletal or mechanical pain and may result from the intervertebral disc, sacroiliac joints, facet joint and muscles. Only a small percentage of cases (5%) are due to nerve root pain, which gives a dermatomal well-localized pain (often with accompanying paraesthesiae). This is usually caused by posterior disc herniation or spinal stenosis. The latter arises as a result of ligament and/or bony hypertrophy of either the spinal canal (central stenosis) or laterally (intervertebral foramina) and typically causes neurogenic claudication after walking. Whilst the overwhelming majority of back pain is not serious, central disc prolapse (causing sphincter disturbance and saddle anaesthesia) requires urgent neurosurgical intervention. Pain associated with serious trauma, suspected malignancy (e.g. associated with weight loss, previous malignancy) or infection will also require rapid investigation.

Patients may need appropriate imaging (plain X rays, CT, MRI). Treatment for mechanical back pain involves NSAIDs together with input from physiotherapy and sometimes clinical psychology. The use of anticonvulsants and antidepressants may be useful if there is evidence of neuropathic pain. In other cases facet joint injection or radiofrequency denervation may provide relief. Epidural steroids may help in early nerve root pain. Other techniques, such as TENS and acupuncture, may be used. Finally, surgery for nerve root pain from anatomically proven disc prolapse or spinal stenosis may also be required.

Neck pain

Neck pain may result from cervical spine degeneration or nerve root compression from cervical disc prolapse and may require surgical intervention. Occipital neuralgia (from C2 root) may require cryotherapy.

Fibromyalgia (FMS) and myofascial (MFS) syndromes

These are two distinct entities of muscle pain.
- FMS is a generalized and widespread pain. It is associated with sleep disorders and psychological problems and may respond to antidepressant medication, fitness training and cognitive behavioural therapy (CBT).
- MFS is a localized muscle pain often associated with a trigger point; palpation causes severe and radiating pain. Localized therapy is useful, such as ultrasound, stretching or injections of local anaesthetic, steroid or botulinum toxin. Other therapies, such as CBT, may also be useful.

Headache and facial pain

There are a number of causes (Table 15.3).

Table 15.3 Causes of headache and facial pain

Migraine
Tension headache
Cluster headaches (and other autonomic headaches)
Temporomandibular joint disorders
Trigeminal neuralgia
Idiopathic facial pain
Postherpetic neuralgia

Figure 16.1 The airway

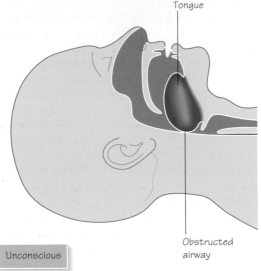

Following sedation/induction of anaesthesia, obstruction can occur from relaxation of the tongue and pharyngeal musculature

Tongue

Unconscious

Obstructed airway

Figure 16.2 Mallampati classification

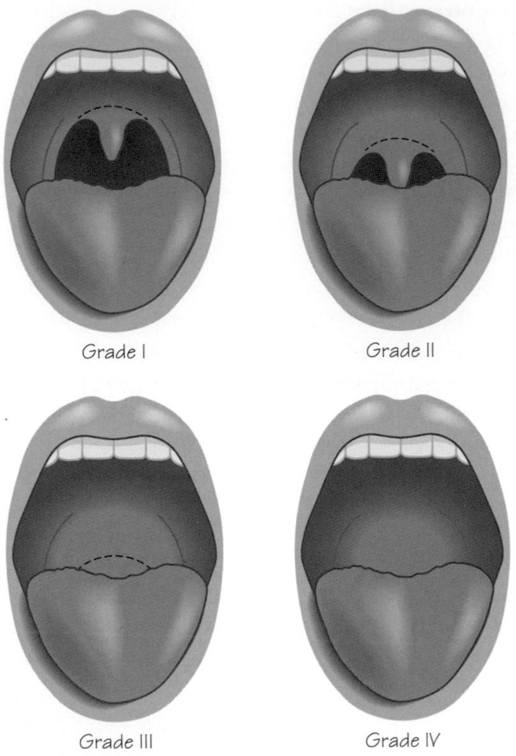

Grade I

Grade II

Grade III

Grade IV

Table 16.1 Techniques used to manage the airway

Technique	Advantage	Disadvantage
Facemask	• Simple	• Difficult for prolonged IPPV • Anaesthetist's hands occupied • No airway protection
Laryngeal mask airway (LMA)	• Simple • Anaesthetist's hands freed up	• May be appropriate for moderate periods of IPPV • Some airway protection • May dislodge
Tracheal tube	• Anaesthetists hand freed up • For IPPV • Usually very secure • Superlative airway protection • Permits IPPV even with stiff lungs/narrowed lower airways	• Requires training • Damage to teeth/airway • Laryngospasm • Prolonged, unrecognized misplacement usually catastrophic

Table 16.2 Reasons for tracheal intubation

	Examples
For paralysis and intermittent positive pressure ventilation (IPPV)	Abdominal/thoracic surgery, head injury, respiratory failure (ICU)
To secure the airway	Partial airway obstruction, shared airway with surgeon
To protect the airway	Blood, gastric contents

Maintaining the airway is the most fundamental aspect of clinical anaesthetic practice. Failure to do so, and the concomitant hypoxia, is still a significant cause of death from anaesthesia. No patient should receive GA or sedation without prior assessment of the airway. During anaesthesia and sedation there is muscular relaxation of the pharynx, which may lead to airway obstruction (Figure 16.1).

In addition, many of the drugs used will cause respiration to cease. Ensuring adequate oxygenation is the priority at all times. Many, but not all, difficult airways may be anticipated in advance.

A separate area is that of the unstable neck, whereby manipulation of the neck may put the patient at risk of spinal cord injury.

Anaesthesia at a Glance, First Edition. Julian Stone and William Fawcett.

Airway assessment

Traditionally, the gold standard of airway management is tracheal intubation, and the majority of assessments relate to the ease or difficulty of this process.

History Ask about:
- past anaesthetic history – see old notes, Medic Alert bracelet;
- surgery/radiotherapy to head and neck;
- obstructive sleep apnoea (OSA);
- conditions affecting tongue size (e.g. acromegaly, infections, tumours);
- conditions affecting neck mobility (e.g. ankylosing spondylitis, infections, tumours);
- conditions affecting mouth opening (e.g. temporamandibular joint dysfunction).

General examination This includes:
- Look for external signs of surgery/radiotherapy to head and neck.
- Assess the airway from in front of the patient, including: receding jaw, protruding upper incisors, large tongue, large neck, obesity.
- Tumours, infection, trauma, swelling or burns and scarring of the airway strongly suggest problems.

Tests A number of tests exist but none are very specific or sensitive. Most attempt to predict the ease of view during subsequent laryngoscopy. These include:
- mouth opening: this should be 4–6 cm;
- Mallampati classification (Figure 16.2): on full opening of the mouth the faucial pillars, uvula and soft palate sequentially disappear; scores of 3 and 4 are associated with difficult intubation;
- forward movement of the jaw, i.e. ability to protrude the lower teeth in front of the upper teeth;
- thyromental distance (chin to thyroid notch): this should be >6 cm;
- sternomental distance (chin to sternum): this should be >12.5 cm;
- atlanto-occipital mobility: this is difficult to assess;
- radiological imaging by CT/MRI.

Management of the airway (basic)

In general, before attempting to sedate or anaesthetize a patient you will need: oxygen; airway devices (Table 16.1); suction and tipping trolley (in case of vomiting); drugs (resuscitation, atropine, suxamethonium); full monitoring; venous access and a skilled assistant.

Facemask The simplest method is spontaneous ventilation via a facemask. Both hands may be required. After a tight seal has been achieved with the facemask and the reservoir bag is full, a number of adjuncts can be used, including: chin lift, jaw thrust, an oral (Guedel) airway and/or nasal airway. This is the most fundamental skill and should be familiar to all who deal with unconscious patients. Bag and mask ventilation for the apnoeic patient is very similar with the anaesthetist (or an assistant) squeezing the reservoir bag.

Laryngeal mask airway (LMA) These are generally easy to insert, provide a safe and reliable airway for spontaneous ventilation and short episodes of intermittent positive pressure ventilation (IPPV).

Tracheal tube This gives definitive airway control, allowing full protection and IPPV.

The expected difficult airway

Before embarking on anaesthesia/sedation in a patient with a known or suspected difficult airway ask:
- Do you need to give GA – what about a regional technique?
- Do you need tracheal intubation – what about LMA (Table 16.2)?
- If you need intubation, is it safe/appropriate to have a look?

Experienced senior help will be required. Be prepared for other adjuncts to tracheal intubation including:
- Fibre-optic intubation, in which the larynx is visualized and then a tube railroaded over the top of the 'scope. This is a very useful technique and can be performed with the patient awake or asleep. With the patient awake the airway is maintained at all times. The airway needs prior preparation (local anaesthesia and nasal vasoconstriction). Any blood in the airway may make this difficult.
- The intubating laryngeal mask airway (ILMA) provides a technique whereby a tracheal tube is inserted down the inside of the LMA.
- Blind nasal intubation is a technique whereby a tracheal tube is passed through the nose and into the trachea without the use of a laryngoscope. It has largely been replaced by fibre-optic intubation.
- Other equipment, such as bougies, may help in the correct placement of a tracheal tube at laryngoscopy.

'Can't intubate, can't ventilate scenario' surgical airway (**cricothyroid puncture/tracheostomy**). Surgical access to the airway, in extremis, is lifesaving. For some operations (e.g. large upper airway cancers) a tracheostomy under local anaesthesia may be performed electively and safely at the start of the procedure (see also Chapter 4).

The unexpected difficult airway

This requires rapid decision making. Oxygenation is again the priority at all times and bag and mask ventilation should proceed whilst a number of choices are considered, depending on the urgency of surgery and the condition of the patient:
- Should surgery proceed? Sometimes the patient may be woken up and the case performed under regional anaesthesia.
- Can the case proceed with bag and mask/LMA?
- Should further attempts at intubation be attempted fibre-optically/ILMA?
- Is a surgical airway required?

Unstable neck

Some patients will have neck pathology whereby the positioning of the head may put the patient at risk of spinal cord damage from unstable cervical vertebrae. Such conditions include trauma, Down syndrome and rheumatoid arthritis. Very careful assessment and stabilization of the neck is required in these cases.

Key points

- The overriding concern is to ensure oxygenation at all times.
- Ensure correct placement of the airway device and monitor this throughout the procedure.
- Never try equipment in an emergency that you are unfamiliar with.
- Never paralyse a patient before ascertaining that ventilation of the lungs via a facemask is possible.
- However daunting it may seem, surgical access to the airway should be considered early on in difficult airway cases.

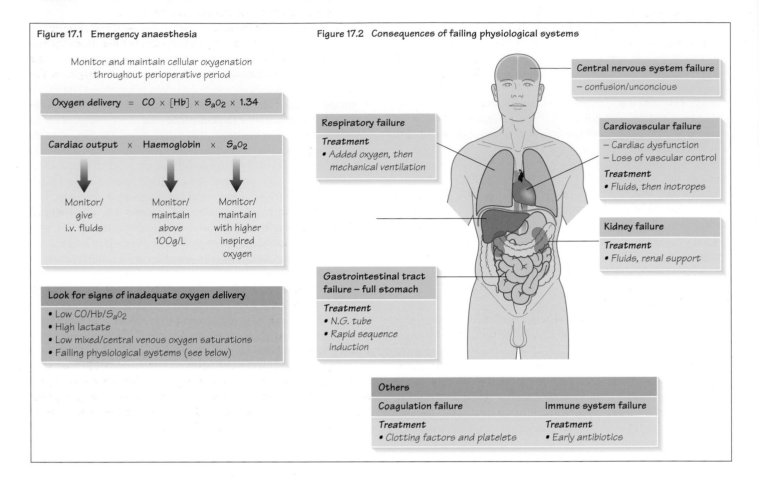

Figure 17.1 Emergency anaesthesia

Figure 17.2 Consequences of failing physiological systems

What is an emergency?

NCEPOD (National Confidential Enquiry into Patient Outcome and Death) defines surgical categories as immediate, urgent, expedited and elective (see Table 6.1).

Pathophysiologies that may be involved include:

- blood loss, e.g. trauma, GI bleeding, postoperative bleeding;
- dehydration, e.g. peritonitis, severe vomiting and diarrhoea;
- sepsis from any cause.

Resuscitation

There is a much higher morbidity and mortality in patients undergoing major emergency surgery in whom preoperative resuscitation is incomplete. Although a few operations ('immediate' cases) require surgery before resuscitation, in the vast majority of cases resuscitation can and should be completed prior to surgery. Three areas have to be considered:

1 the patient's underlying co-morbidity;
2 the presenting problem and its physiological sequelae;
3 the magnitude of surgery contemplated.

In general, it may be difficult to radically change underlying co-morbidity (e.g. ischaemic heart disease/COPD) in the limited time frame, although some improvements may be possible. The major focus therefore is correcting physiological upset. Generally, this involves correcting fluid/blood loss associated with the problem (e.g. from gastrointestinal losses or blood loss, especially in trauma) and for some patients prolonged dehydration due to gastrointestinal obstruction. Occasionally, lesser surgery may have to be undertaken if the patient's condition is too poor.

Signs of an adequately resuscitated patient

1 **Clinical:**

(a) cardiovascular: adequate blood pressure and heart rate (as a guide: systolic >100 mmHg; pulse <100 bpm)
(b) respiratory: respiratory rate <15 breaths/min
(c) kidney: adequate urine output of at least 0.5 mL/kg/h;
(d) CNS: a poorly resuscitated patients may be drowsy or even unconscious.

These are only guides; for example the patient may be beta blocked and therefore unable mount a tachycardia, or they may have received opioids so that the respiratory rate is reduced.

2 **Cardiovascular monitoring:**

(a) Central venous pressure (CVP): for some patients this provides a valuable guide to fluid replacement. CVP approximates to ventricular end diastolic pressure and hence to preload. Normal pressure is 4–8 mmHg. Low pressures indicate that further fluids should be administered, whereas high pressures suggest that adequate or

Anaesthesia at a Glance, First Edition. Julian Stone and William Fawcett.

excess fluids have been given or that other problems such as cardiac failure are present.

(b) Cardiac output measurements: various estimations are made from Doppler measurements (see Figure 5.2) or by wave form analysis from arterial cannulae. This allows stroke volume to be calculated and again the response to fluid challenges can be assessed.

3 Biochemical monitoring: various indices of adequate perfusion and oxygenation have been used (Figure 17.1):

(a) Arterial blood gas analysis: a metabolic acidosis is a common. A base excess of −5 mmol/L indicates a moderate acidosis and a base excess of −10 mmol/L indicates a severe acidosis, which would necessitate the patient receiving intensive care postoperatively, perhaps for ventilation.

(b) Lactate concentration: a lactate of over 2 mmol/L implies significant anaerobic metabolism; greater than 4 mmol/L suggests serious metabolic derangement.

(c) Central venous oxygen saturation ($S_{cv}O_2$): this may reflect mixed venous oxygenation, itself an indicator of oxygen extraction. Low levels (<70%) imply inadequate cardiac output with excessive oxygen extraction in the tissues.

Gastric emptying

Beware of the full stomach! Elective surgery differs from emergency surgery in that the former almost always takes place with an empty stomach. As a result, protection of the airway from stomach contents with a cuffed tracheal tube is not commonly necessary. Conversely, emergency patients very often have to be considered as having a full stomach. Reasons for this include (see Figure 6.2):

- time from last meal may be less than 6 hours;
- failure of the stomach to empty due to;
  - any significant intra-abdominal pathology, e.g. peritonitis;
  - gastrointestinal obstruction;
  - administration of opioids;
  - multiply injured patients.

Preparing a patient for emergency surgery

The usual history and examination should be carried out. Investigations will usually include haemoglobin, U&E, blood clotting and group, and save serum (or cross match). Determination of arterial blood gases for base excess and lactate should be considered. For the sickest patients, induction of anaesthesia in theatre and not the anaesthetic room may be appropriate.

Patients scheduled for major surgery will need (Figure 17.2):
- Higher inspired oxygen.
- Venous access for i.v. fluids, including blood and blood products; one or two large peripheral cannulae are required.
- Some will need CVP monitoring to facilitate fluid management.
- Blood transfusion may be required. Remember that haemoglobin may be normal/high due to haemoconcentration but anaemia may be unmasked following resuscitation. Haemoglobin of 100 g/L is the lowest desirable.
- Analgesia: regional blockade such as epidural may be contraindicated in this scenario for a number of reasons:
  - hypovolaemia/hypotension;
  - coagulopathy;
  - sepsis;
  - neurological injury;
  - problems with positioning of the patient;
  - may be inappropriate, e.g. when the patient is due for prolonged ventilation postoperatively.
- Temperature control
- Urinary catheter
- Antibiotics
- Many gastrointestinal emergencies will need nasogastric tubes to decompress stomach.
- Risks of surgery need to be discussed with patient and/or family.

Postoperative care

Patients may deteriorate postoperatively, requiring ventilation, inotropic support, renal replacement therapy, etc. The markers used preoperatively for resuscitation are useful postoperatively. The appropriate level of care needs to be arranged, such as intensive care or high dependency. In addition, patients will require:
- oxygen;
- i.v. fluids;
- medication alternatives if still nil by mouth;
- thromboprophylaxis.

Patients in extremis

Occasionally, patients present very late and/or with no time for resuscitation and the situation demands immediate surgery. The same principles apply but the patients may need in addition the presence of inotropes and a defibrillator in theatre. In addition, they may need O negative or group specific uncrossmatched blood and treatment of severe acidosis with sodium bicarbonate.

Figure 18.1 Physiological changes during pregnancy

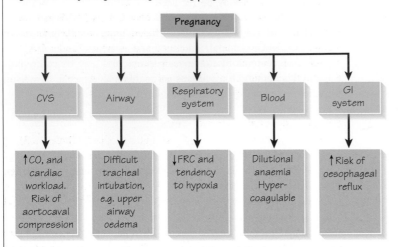

Figure 18.2 Anatomy relevant to spinal and epidural anaesthesia

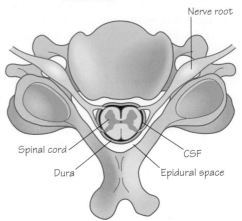

Table 18.1 Problems with regional blockade

- Hypotension (i.v. access mandatory)
- Weakness (even with 'mobile mixtures')
- Post dural puncture headache
- Prolongation of labour
- Neurological damage (<1:10,000)

Table 18.3 Contraindications to regional blockade

- Patient refusal
- No i.v. access
- Allergy to amide local anaesthetics
- Sepsis
- Coagulopathy
- Cardiovascular – hypovolaemia and severe cardiac disease, e.g. stenotic valvular disease
- Major spinal surgery, e.g. spinal rods

Figure 18.3 Effects of injecting local anaesthetic drugs into the epidural space

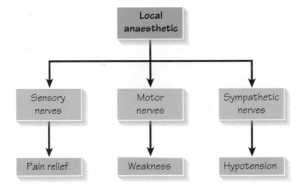

Table 18.4 Leading causes of death in obstetrics

- Sepsis
- Thrombosis and thromboembolism
- Pre-eclampsia and eclampsia
- Haemorrhage
- Amniotic fluid embolism

Table 18.2 Comparison of epidural and spinal anaesthesia

Epidural (or extradural)	Spinal (or intrathecal)
• Catheter inserted therefore can be topped up	• 'Single shot' into CSF (so cannot be topped up)
• Slow onset	• Rapid onset
• Large needle	• Small needle
• For labour analgesia/LSCS/instrumental	• LSCS/instrumental/retained placenta
• May get missed segments	• Missed segments rare

Anaesthesia at a Glance, First Edition. Julian Stone and William Fawcett.

Many of the physiological changes that take place in pregnancy are of relevance to all obstetric anaesthesia (Figure 18.1). There are a variety of methods of pain relief in labour (e.g. TENS, entonox and pethidine) that are provided without anaesthetic input. Methods with anaesthetic input are described in this chapter.

Epidurals for pain relief in labour

Epidurals provide excellent segmental analgesia. The anatomy of the spinal and epidural spaces is shown in Figure 18.2.

What solution is used in the epidural?

Local anaesthetics (LA) were used on their own for many years. The effects of injecting local anaesthetic drugs in to the epidural space is shown in Figure 18.3. Bupivacaine is the only LA used as it is long acting and has low transfer to the fetus. Some of the side effects, particularly leg weakness, can be reduced by adding an opioid (commonly fentanyl) to the LA, which also enhances analgesia. This LA/ opioid mixture was popularized as the mobile epidural.

What are the side effects/risks? (Table 18.1, Figure 18.3)

- Hypotension from sympathetic block.
- Weakness (much less with mobile mixtures).
- Urinary retention may occur.
- Headache from accidental dural puncture, which has an incidence of about 0.6%. The resultant CSF leak causes a severe headache, which will often require a blood patch – a repeat epidural injection at a later date in which blood is injected.
- Catheter misplacement so that the injectate goes not into the epidural space but into the CSF or intravenously. The former will cause a total spinal anaesthesia from head to toe, together with total paralysis and loss of consciousness. The latter will cause cardiac arrhythmias which are often refractory to treatment, although L-bupivacaine is a safer isomer than the standard racemic mixture of the two isomers, and is becoming the drug of choice.
- Neurological damage: although very rare this can occur because of direct trauma to the nervous tissue, injecting the wrong substance or because of a space-occupying lesion in the vertebral canal (from either blood or an abscess) compressing the spinal cord. An epidural catheter must therefore only be sited in the absence of coagulopathy and infection.
- Duration of labour may be increased.
- Regional techniques do not cause backache.

Lower segment Caesarean section

Some 20% of deliveries will require lower segment Caesarean section (LSCS). If possible a regional technique is preferred. Patients should always have a full blood count and be grouped and saved. O negative blood should always be on hand for very urgent resuscitation.

Patients should receive antacid prophylaxis, usually H_2 antagonists and 30 mL 0.3 M sodium citrate. The risk of aortocaval compression (with the pregnant uterus preventing venous return and compressing the aorta, causing hypotension and a marked reduction in cardiac output) should be minimized with a left lateral tilt/wedge. In addition, the position of the placenta should be known as low-lying anterior placentae may be associated with massive blood loss.

LSCS – regional anaesthesia

Regional anaesthesia is preferred to general anaesthesia as it is safer for the mother and the baby compared to GA. If the patient has an indwelling and effective epidural catheter then this can be topped up and used for the surgery. This will take around 20 minutes to become effective. If no epidural catheter is *in situ* then a single shot spinal is often preferred as the regional technique of choice as it is quick and relatively simple. It will last for 1–1.5 hours. A comparison of epidural and spinal anaesthesia is show in Table 18.2.

The benefits of regional anaesthesia over GA for LSCS include:
- avoidance of the risks of GA – failed intubation, aspiration of stomach contents, neonatal depression and awareness under GA;
- good analgesia immediately postoperatively;
- possible reduction in blood loss and pulmonary thromboembolism;
- usually a positive experience for both mother and partner.

LSCS – general anaesthesia

Sometimes a regional technique is contraindicated (Table 18.3) or there is insufficient time. A GA carries much greater risk in late pregnancy, with increased risk of difficult/failed tracheal intubation, hypoxia and aspiration of gastric contents. A GA must therefore take place only with skilled assistance, a tipping table and good suction.

One or two peripheral cannulae, antacid prophylaxis, preoxygenation and full monitoring are required. Rapid sequence induction of anaesthesia and cricoid pressure is mandatory. A variety of airway devices (including tracheal tubes, introducers, laryngeal mask and cricothyroidotomy set) must always be at hand.

Failed tracheal intubation should be prepared for. All departments have a protocol for this, which includes either waking the patient up, or, if urgent, continuing with a GA in the absence of a tracheal tube, e.g. with an LMA instead.

Other areas

Pre-eclampsia, eclampsia and HELLP syndrome

Pre-eclampsia (hypertension, oedema and proteinuria) may worsen to severe pre-eclampsia with headaches, epigastric pain and pulmonary oedema and HELLP syndrome (haemolysis, elevated liver enzymes and low platelets) and result in eclamptic convulsions. This requires:
- airway and oxygenation;
- control of convulsions (i.v. magnesium);
- fluid balance, including administration of blood products;
- awareness of platelet and coagulation studies if regional anaesthesia contemplated;
- risks of general anaesthesia if contemplated, especially cerebral haemorrhage (e.g. due to hypertensive surge on laryngoscopy) and failed intubation.

Haemorrhage

Massive haemorrhage may be occult (no external bleeding). Basic signs (e.g. tachycardia and hypotension) should alert staff to blood loss with the rapid institution of good i.v. access (including CVP) line and blood products (including O negative blood).

Risks

For the last 60 years a triennial report has produced data on every obstetric death in the UK. The current organization is called MBRRACE-UK (Mothers and Babies – Reducing Risk through Audits and Confidential Enquiries across the UK). Leading causes of obstetric deaths are given in Table 18.4. In spite of improvements in anaesthetic safety, anaesthesia still remains a significant cause of death during childbirth.

19 Ophthalmic anaesthesia

Figure 19.1 Intraocular pressure–volume relationship and 'compliance'

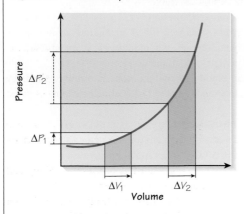

At lower volumes a small increase in volume ΔV_1, causes only small increase in pressure ΔP_1

At higher volumes a small increase in volume ΔV_2, causes a **marked** increase in pressure ΔP_2

Figure 19.2 Causes of raised intraocular pressure

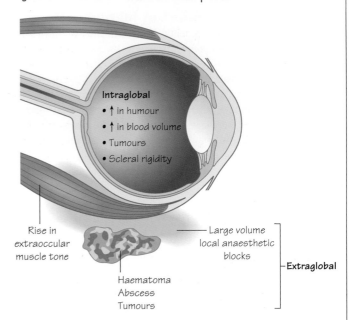

Intraglobal
- ↑ in humour
- ↑ in blood volume
- Tumours
- Scleral rigidity

Rise in extraoccular muscle tone

Haematoma
Abscess
Tumours

Large volume local anaesthetic blocks

Extraglobal

Table 19.1 Avoidance of rises in intraocular pressure

Control blood volume	• Avoid high arterial pressure, e.g. at intubation
	• Avoid high venous pressure:
	  – no coughing
	  – head up
	  – unobstructed neck veins
	• Intermittent positive pressure ventilation to control $PaCO_2$

Control extraocular muscle tone	• Avoid suxamethonium • Good muscle relaxation
Avoid global compression	• Avoid large volumes of local anaesthetic • Avoid facemask pressure
Reduce aqueous production	• Acetazolamide • Mannitol

Table 19.2 Local anaesthetic techniques in ophthalmic surgery

	Topical	Peribulbar	Sub-Tenon's block	Retrobulbar
Advantages	• Easy, very safe	• Good anaesthesia and akinesia	• Safe • Good anaesthesia and akinesia	• Good anaesthesia and akinesia
Disadvantages	• No akinesia	• Globe penetration • Haemorrhage • Muscle damage • Inadvertent i.v. injection	• Conjunctival haemorrhage	• Globe penetration • Haemorrhage • Muscle damage • Optic nerve damage/ penetration • Facial nerve block required • Inadvertent i.v. injection

Anaesthesia at a Glance, First Edition. Julian Stone and William Fawcett.

Anaesthesia for ophthalmic surgery can be divided into the following areas:
- cataract surgery (usually elderly);
- squint surgery (usually children);
- corneal and vitreoretinal surgery;
- emergency surgery.

A key area in ophthalmic anaesthesia involves the factors that increase or lower intraocular pressure (IOP). The eye (like the brain) is a rigid structure that has very little ability to expand, therefore any increase in intraocular volume rapidly causes a marked increase in IOP. This pressure–volume or compliance relationship is shown in Figure 19.1.

The normal IOP is 10–20 mmHg. A rise in IOP from intraglobal causes (e.g. blood, aqueous) or from extrinsic pressure can cause IOP to rise to dangerous levels. In an intact eye, perfusion of the retina is put at risk if IOP exceeds retinal artery pressure. However, should a rise in IOP occur when the eye is open during surgery or during a penetrating eye injury it may cause the loss of intraorbital contents (e.g. vitreous/lens) etc. The factors that cause a raised IOP are shown in Figure 19.2. Preventing a rise in IOP is fundamental to good ophthalmic anaesthesia and strategies are shown in Table 19.1.

Cataract surgery

The essential requirements are anaesthesia of the conjunctiva together with a quiet eye, that is no rise in intraocular pressure. Some surgeons require akinesia too, necessitating additional anaesthesia to topical (surface) anaesthesia. The majority of these procedures are carried out under local anaesthesia, with patients spending only a couple of hours in hospital. There are a number of available techniques (Table 19.2).

1 Topical anaesthesia alone, e.g. oxybuprocaine.

2 Sub-Tenon's block (episcleral) in which, after making a small incision in the inferonasal portion of the conjunctiva and Tenon's capsule, and undertaking a little blunt dissection, the local anaesthetic is injected using a blunt needle.

3 Peribulbar block: a 25-mm, 25-G needle is used to inject outside the extraocular muscle cone. Usually an inferotemporal injection is used, supplemented if required by a medial injection.

4 Retrobulbar block (which is almost obsolete): the injection requires instillation within the muscle cone. Very often, a supplementary facial nerve block is also required.

Intravenous access, pulse oximetry and ECG are often used for techniques 2–4. Occasionally sedation is used (e.g. small increments of midazolam 1 mg).

Complications of local anaesthetic techniques are usually due to sharp needle damage (techniques 3 and 4) and include:
- retrobulbar haemorrhage;
- globe penetration: this is more likely in a myopic eye with a long axial length (>26 mm) and will often cause a vitreous haemorrhage and blindness;
- injection into muscle (paresis) or into the optic nerve (blindness) or around the nerve where it can track along the dura of the optic nerve to cause a total spinal anaesthetic (resulting in apnoea and loss of consciousness);
- intravenous injection.

Contraindications to local anaesthesia are:
- refusal by the patient, or they are unable to lie flat or still;
- INR >2.5 for techniques 2–4.

If a general anaesthetic is required then attempts are made to provide a low IOP with moderate hyperventilation. The airway may be secured with a tracheal tube or laryngeal mask.

Squint surgery

This is usually undertaken on children under general anaesthetic. There are a number of issues.
- The airway is covered by drapes and needs to be secured either by a LMA, or in small children (<2 years old) a tracheal tube is often preferred.
- The oculocardiac reflex: pressure/tension on the globe or eye muscles can cause a marked bradycardia, which can be avoided by pretreatment with atropine.
- There is a high incidence of postoperative nausea and vomiting and pretreatment with an antiemetic is usually advisable.
- Suxamethonium is best avoided as this is a trigger for malignant hyperthermia (MH); there is a higher incidence of MH in patients undergoing squint surgery.

Vitreoretinal surgery

Patients often have had retinal detachments and/or vitreous haemorrhage. Co-morbidities are common and include diabetes (and all its attendant complications). Gas may be injected into the eye during the operation; N_2O may have to be avoided (as it expands gas-filled spaces) and the patient may have to lie in a certain position postoperatively. Laser is sometimes used, necessitating theatre staff to wear goggles. To prevent the oculocardiac reflex the afferent limb of the reflex arc can be blocked with local anaesthetic or pretreatment with atropine.

Penetrating eye injury

The major issue here is that IOP has to be controlled until the surgery is complete, as the risk is expulsion of the intraocular contents and blindness. If the patient is not adequately fasted, then two opposing factors have to be reconciled:
- Is it better to secure the airway using suxamethonium and a rapid sequence induction, and risk a rise in IOP (see Chapter 12)?
- Or is it better to avoid suxamethonium and use a non-depolarizing agent, which has greater risk to the airway?

There is no right answer. Whilst the airway is more precious than the eye, if the anaesthetist is confident of his/her ability to successfully undertake tracheal intubation without suxamethonium then many would choose that option. If so and a non-depolarizing agent is used, neuromuscular monitoring must be in place as attempted intubation and laryngoscopy and intubation without full paralysis is every bit as harmful to IOP as the use of suxamethonium.

Problems in ophthalmic anaesthesia

The two main problems encountered in ophthalmic anaesthesia are:
1 The airway not readily accessible as it is covered by drapes. This is of relevance with both LAs, GAs and sedation.
2 The theatre may be in subdued lighting, adding to the above risk.

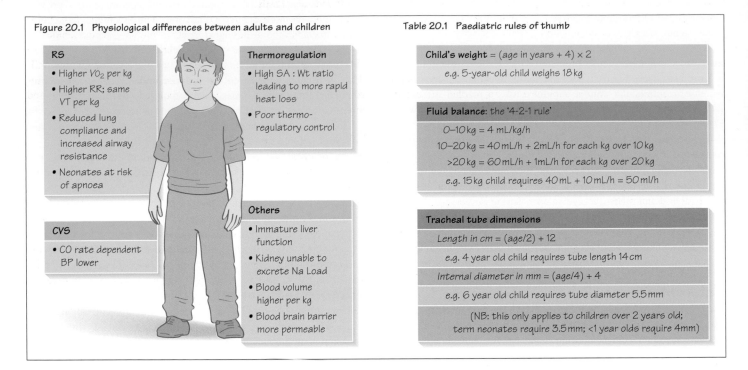

Figure 20.1 Physiological differences between adults and children

RS
- Higher VO_2 per kg
- Higher RR; same VT per kg
- Reduced lung compliance and increased airway resistance
- Neonates at risk of apnoea

CVS
- CO rate dependent BP lower

Thermoregulation
- High SA : Wt ratio leading to more rapid heat loss
- Poor thermo-regulatory control

Others
- Immature liver function
- Kidney unable to excrete Na Load
- Blood volume higher per kg
- Blood brain barrier more permeable

Table 20.1 Paediatric rules of thumb

Child's weight = (age in years + 4) × 2
e.g. 5-year-old child weighs 18 kg

Fluid balance: the '4-2-1 rule'

0–10 kg = 4 mL/kg/h
10–20 kg = 40 mL/h + 2 mL/h for each kg over 10 kg
>20 kg = 60 mL/h + 1 mL/h for each kg over 20 kg
e.g. 15 kg child requires 40 mL + 10 mL/h = 50 ml/h

Tracheal tube dimensions

Length in cm = (age/2) + 12
e.g. 4 year old child requires tube length 14 cm
Internal diameter in mm = (age/4) + 4
e.g. 6 year old child requires tube diameter 5.5 mm
(NB: this only applies to children over 2 years old; term neonates require 3.5 mm; <1 year olds require 4 mm)

Anaesthetic management of children

There are a number of differences between adults and children, and in particular neonates (Figure 20.1). Children are not just miniature adults; their body parts have different proportions and their organs are less mature. These differences are most marked in neonates and become less distinct as children get older.

Preoperative assessment

Rapport should be established with the child and his/her parent(s) and a parent should be invited to the anaesthetic room.

Note is made of weight and age, including prematurity. Much of the adult preassessment template may be used, such as previous illnesses, medication and allergies, and teeth. In addition, upper respiratory tract infections (URTIs) are not uncommon in young children and place the child at increased risk of perioperative respiratory problems. Ideally, several weeks should have elapsed following a URTI, although some children have recurrent URTIs and it may not be practical to delay surgery. However, any child with a productive cough, chest signs or a temperature should not be submitted to elective surgery.

Preoperative tests are seldom required, especially for healthy children undergoing minor surgery.

A plan of the anaesthetic should be discussed with the parents and includes the method of induction, postoperative analgesia (including the use of suppositories) and what to expect in terms of i.v. cannulae, infusions, nasogastric tubes, etc.

Fasting for children will be in line with local policy and is typically 2 hours for clear fluids and 6 hours for solids (as in adults). Fasting times for milk is generally taken to be 4 hours, although some advocate only 3 hours for breast milk.

Premedication is usually topical local anaesthetic for venous access. Some centres administer routine preoperative analgesia (e.g. a loading dose of paracetamol) and care needs to be taken that another dose is not inadvertently administered.

Induction of anaesthesia

As in adults, anaesthesia can be induced intravenously or by inhalation. If i.v. access is already present, this is usually employed. Intravenous access may be challenging as the veins may be small, poorly visible (especially in 6–18 month olds) due to subcutaneous fat and of course painful even with topical anaesthetic. Inhalational induction requires the ability to minimize entrainment of air and allow high concentrations of anaesthetic to reach the alveoli. The combination of sevoflurane and nitrous oxide in oxygen is very potent, rapid and smooth.

Maintenance of anaesthesia

This is almost always inhalational as i.v. techniques (e.g. propofol) are not licensed in young children. Spontaneously breathing techniques are suitable for older children and/or short procedures. In very young children (infants) the additional work of breathing through the tracheal tube necessitates artificial ventilation of the lungs in all but the very shortest procedures.

Reversal of anaesthesia

Neuromuscular blockade is reversed in the same way as in adults.

Areas of interest
The airway

Securing the airway is fundamental for all anaesthetics. If the child has undergone inhalational induction, it is essential that no attempt is made to instrument the airway (e.g. laryngoscopy, tracheal intubation, insertion of LMA) until venous access is secured as laryngospasm may result. A Guedel airway may be inserted. If laryngeal spasm does occur without venous access, suxamethonium can be given i.m. (or some administer it sublingually). The narrowest part of the airway is just below the vocal cords. Selection of tracheal tube size is important (Table 20.1). If there is no audible leak around the tube then it may be too tight, leading to postextubation oedema and stridor.

Pain control

Assessment of pain control is fundamental postoperatively. Depending on the magnitude of surgery, a number of approaches should be considered.

Paracetamol A loading dose of is often given on the ward, followed by regular postoperative doses.

NSAIDs Diclofenac (per rectum) is useful and often administered under general anaesthesia after obtaining parental consent.

Opioids These are best avoided via the i.m. route and can be intravenously administered in the older child as patient-controlled analgesia (PCA) or nurse-controlled analgesia (NCA) in the younger child.

Local anaesthesia This can be administered into the wound or via nerve blocks. Caudals are commonly used for pelvic operations but epidurals and other nerve blocks are less common outside of specialist centres.

Intravenous fluids

The use of hypotonic solutions for maintenance fluids (e.g. 0.4% dextrose, 0.18% saline) for children is not routinely recommended as this may lead to hyponatraemia and cerebral oedema. Most would give either 0.9% saline or Hartmann's solution. For resuscitation of children, up to 20 mL/kg of colloid may be used as a bolus. Glucose-containing solutions are not usually required except in babies and those with hypoglycaemia.

Thermoregulation

Young children and babies are at risk of hypothermia and, in general, warming of theatres and i.v. fluid with temperature monitoring are vital.

Drug handling

There are pharmacodynamic and pharmacokinetic differences in neonates and babies, leading to altered drug effects. These include increased opioid and neuromuscular sensitivity (pharmacodynamic) and increased volume of distribution (pharmacokinetic) of suxamethonium.

Figure 21.1 Front view of coronary artery bypass graft (CABG)

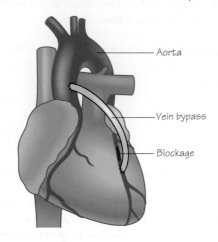

- Aorta
- Vein bypass
- Blockage

Figure 21.2 Cardiopulmonary bypass machine

- Aortic cannula
- Filter
- Cardiotomy suction device
- SVC
- Roller pump
- Venous cannula
- Gas flow
- Reservoir
- Oxygenator
- IVC
- Heat exchanger

Table 21.1 Determinants of myocardial supply and demand

Supply increased by increased:	• Coronary perfusion pressure (DAP – LVEDP) • Diastolic time (i.e. bradycardia) • Vessel wall diameter
Demand increased by increased:	• SAP • Heart rate • Myocardial contractility

DAP, diastolic arterial pressure; LVEDP, left ventricular end diastolic pressure; SAP, systolic arterial pressure

Table 21.2 Adverse effects of cardiopulmonary bypass

- Systemic inflammatory response syndrome (SIRS)
- Platelet dysfunction
- Clotting disorders: fibrinolysis and consumptive coagulopathy
- Haemolysis
- Neurological injury: stroke and psychological/ psychiatric changes (from emboli)
- Renal injury

Figure 21.3 Double-lumen tube in situ

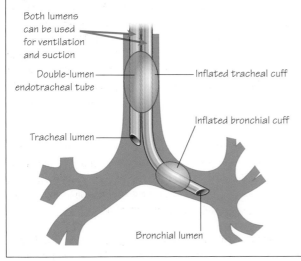

- Both lumens can be used for ventilation and suction
- Double-lumen endotracheal tube
- Tracheal lumen
- Inflated tracheal cuff
- Inflated bronchial cuff
- Bronchial lumen

Table 21.3 Methods of pain control after thoracotomy

Technique	Comments
Systemic opioids, e.g. PCA	• May cause respiratory and cough depression • Some add ketamine to the opioid
Epidural analgesia	• Excellent analgesia but may cause hypotension and intercostal muscle block
Paravertebral block	• Avoids hypotension and can be used with other techniques, e.g. PCA
Interpleural block	• Effective but solution can be lost through chest drains
Intrathecal opioids, e.g. morphine	• Effective but single shot • Potential for delayed respiratory depression

PCA, patient-controlled analgesia

Cardiac anaesthesia

The majority of cardiac anaesthesia involves anaesthetizing for either coronary artery bypass surgery or valve replacement. Coronary disease is the major cause of death in the western world. In general, patients with symptomatic disease may undergo pharmacological treatment or have the atheroma within the coronary arteries managed by cardiologists (percutaneous coronary intervention [PCI]), with angioplasty (with or without stents) or undergo open surgery (coronary artery bypass graft [CABG] surgery; Figure 21.1).

Preoperative preparation

Patients undergoing open heart surgery will have had extensive preoperative investigations for major surgery. In particular, echocardiogra-

Anaesthesia at a Glance, First Edition. Julian Stone and William Fawcett.

phy and left heart catheterization provides information about coronary anatomy, ventricular function and valve gradients.

Peroperative management

Patients undergoing major cardiac surgery will generally have a sedative premedication and have central venous and arterial lines inserted under local anaesthesia prior to induction with full haemodynamic monitoring. Haemodynamic stability is paramount to prevent a rise or fall in blood pressure, both of which may precipitate cardiac ischaemia. The determinants of myocardial blood supply and demand are shown in Table 21.1.

Many patients undergoing cardiac surgery require cardiopulmonary bypass (CPB; Figure 21.2) whereby blood is drained from the venous circulation in large tubes to the CPB machine, where it is oxygenated (via a membrane oxygenator) and pressurized (by means of a roller pump or centrifugal pump) and returned to the aorta. During this time ventilation of the lungs is not required. This process permits the surgeon to operate on a still, bloodless heart. Prior to CPB the patient is anticoagulated with heparin. The patient is cooled to reduce metabolic rate and minimize cardiac (and other organ) damage. When undergoing cardiopulmonary bypass, careful monitoring of coagulation and acid–base balance and an intravenous anaesthetic technique is required.

Once surgery is complete the patient is rewarmed and the heart is restarted. Discontinuation of CPB occurs by diverting more of the venous return to the right heart and the lungs. Once the patient is stable (with or without vasoactive medication), the major vessels are decannulated, the heparinization reversed with protamine and the patient's chest is closed.

CPB is not without major complications (Table 21.2). Some of these changes can be reduced by coating the CPB tubing with heparin and phosphorylcholine, and the use of leucocyte filters to reduce platelet consumption and the systemic inflammatory response syndrome (SIRS). The use of centrifugal pumps may reduce haemolysis.

Other techniques used for cardiac surgery include deep hypothermic circulatory arrest (DHCA) to protect the brain, which is often used in paediatric or aortic surgery. The patient is cooled to 18°C and up to 30 min of DCHA is usually tolerated. The patient receives further neuroprotection from i.v. anaesthetics and strict glycaemic control. Another technique is off-pump coronary artery surgery, which was developed in an attempt to limit the adverse effects of CPB.

Postoperative management

The patient is ventilated until stable in terms of cardiac function, gas exchange, metabolic function, blood loss and temperature, and then extubated. Vasoactive drugs may be required to control blood pressure and cardiac output. Blood loss is carefully monitored and coagulopathy treated as required. Rapid bleeding and especially cardiac tamponade (rising CVP and falling blood pressure) will necessitate a prompt return to theatre.

Thoracic surgery

Thoracic surgery is arguably one of the most challenging areas in anaesthesia. It commonly involves surgery on the lungs and pleura (tumours and infection) or the oesophagus.

A major requirement for thoracic surgery is to be able to treat the left and right lung as two separate structures, being ventilated and protected (from blood/secretions) independently. The standard tracheal tube is not usually sufficient and a double-lumen tube (DLT; Figures 4.4 and 21.3) is employed, with one lumen opening into the trachea and one opening into a main bronchus. There are two cuffs on the tube, thus both lungs can be isolated from each other.

Management of patients undergoing major thoracic surgery

Preoperative management

Patients will require comprehensive assessment of their respiratory function and reserve, particularly if they are scheduled to have a lung resection, as it must be ascertained that the remaining lung tissue is adequate for ventilatory exchange and coughing. Patients will require baseline chest X ray, and arterial blood gas analysis and respiratory function tests, often including cardiopulmonary exercise testing (CPET).

Prior to surgery, the patient may require optimization of respiratory function (including cessation of smoking) and many patients undergoing oesophageal resection will require nutritional support, including enteral feeding by means of a jejunostomy.

Peroperative management

Patients require full vascular (arterial and central) access. Challenging areas include:

Double-lumen tube placement These tubes are preformed and made for either passage into the left or right main bronchus. The position of the tube is often verified fibre-optically.

One lung anaesthesia (OLA) During lung resection, and also during oesophageal surgery, the patient's chest is open and the upper lung is not used for ventilation as it obscures access. Therefore all the ventilation is directed to the lower lung. However, although most of the pulmonary blood flow goes to the lower lung some blood still passes through the upper lung, and will not be oxygenated. This ventilation–perfusion (VQ) mismatch causes deoxygenated blood to pass into the systemic circulation and can render the patient markedly hypoxic; intermittent reinflation of the upper lung may have to be used. In addition, there may be postoperative lung dysfunction following OLA.

Pain control after thoracotomy Good postoperative pain control is essential to permit lung expansion and secretion removal (via coughing) as well as mobilization. Some methods are shown in Table 21.3. Balanced (multimodal) analgesia with the use of regular simple analgesics (e.g. paracetamol/NSAIDs) is recommended.

Fluid management Following thoracic surgery, excess fluid may cause an increase in pulmonary complications, whereas too little fluid will reduce cardiac output and oxygen delivery. Many choose relative fluid restriction, with close monitoring, to minimize pulmonary complications.

Figure 22.1 Diagram of a spinal needle entering the cerebrospinal fluid (CSF)

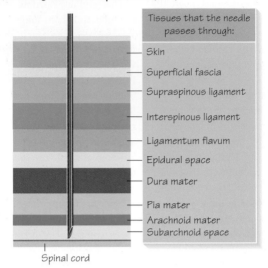

Tissues that the needle passes through:

- Skin
- Superficial fascia
- Supraspinous ligament
- Interspinous ligament
- Ligamentum flavum
- Epidural space
- Dura mater
- Pia mater
- Arachnoid mater
- Subarchnoid space

Spinal cord

Figure 22.2 Ultrasound images to locate targeted nerves

(a) Interscalene view

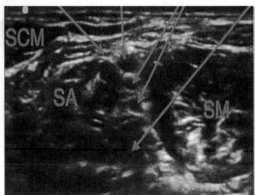

SCM, sternocleidomastoid; SA, scalenus anterior; SM, scalenus medius. Arrows from left to right clockwise: phrenic nerve, C5, C6 (double arrow), C7

(b) Axillary view

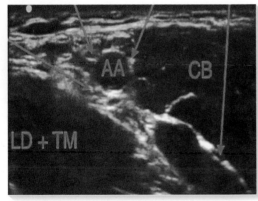

LD, latissimus dorsi; CB, coracobrachialis; AA, axillary artery. Arrows from left to right clockwise: radial nerve, ulnar nerve, median nerve, musculocutaneous nerve

Regional anaesthesia involves the injection of local anaesthetic (LA) and sometimes other drugs (e.g. opioids) targeted at a specific nerve(s) or nerve plexus to numb the area that the nerve innervates, including the spinal cord and its nerve roots. Indications for a nerve block include:
- sole form of anaesthesia during an operation;
- combined with general anaesthesia or sedation;
- postoperative analgesia;
- chronic pain conditions.

Central (neuraxial) blockade
Central blockade is the introduction of drugs into the CSF within the subarachnoid space (spinal blockade; Figure 22.1) or the surrounding epidural space (epidural blockade). Anaesthesia is provided for surgery below the level of the umbilicus (T10).

Advantages of central blockade are:
- avoidance of GA in at-risk patients, e.g. severe respiratory disease, difficult intubation, diabetic, myopathies, pregnant, malignant hyperthermia;
- good postoperative analgesia;
- avoids sedation/nausea and vomiting, e.g. by morphine;
- reduction in pulmonary thromboembolism due to sympathetic block;
- reduced blood loss;
- reduced stress response to surgery.
  Side effects of central blockade are:
- hypotension (sympathetic block);
- nausea and vomiting (hypotension, opiates);
- lower limb motor block;
- post dural puncture headache (more likely with large needle, non-pencil-point tip, inadvertent Tuohy needle puncture of dura, young age);

Anaesthesia at a Glance, First Edition. Julian Stone and William Fawcett.
54

- high block can effect upper limb power and respiration (C3–5);
- loss of consciousness (total spinal);
- nerve damage (rare).

Contraindications to central blockade include patient refusal, no i.v. access, severe CVS disease, hypovolaemia, sepsis, LA allergy, coagulopathy (e.g. INR needs to be <1.5). Caution must be exercised if there has been previous major spinal surgery or ongoing CNS disease.

Spinal block

The spinal cord terminates at the lower border of L1 or upper border of L2. A spinal needle must be introduced at or below the L2/L3 interspace. Tuffier's line is a useful landmark, that is a line drawn between the iliac crests corresponding to the level of L4/5.

Spinal needles are narrow gauged (25 or 27 G) so as to make as small a hole in the dura mater as possible. The most commonly used needle has a blunt 'pencil-point tip', which separates the dural fibres rather than cutting, reducing the incidence of CSF leak-related headache.

To perform a spinal anaesthetic the patient either sits or lies on their side. In both cases their back must be curled forward in order to widen the intervertebral disc spaces. LA ampoules for spinal block often contain dextrose as well, to increase its baricity in relation to the CSF. Once injected, the 'heavy' LA sinks, allowing a denser block on one side if required (e.g. with the patient lying on their side, heavy local anaesthetic will affect the dependent side more). Plain LA is hypobaric and will affect the non-dependent (lower) side more.

A full aseptic technique must be used with gloves, gown, mask and cap.

Epidural block

This involves the placement of a catheter into the epidural space, followed by continuous or intermittent drug administration. It is used for analgesia during labour as well as during surgery and for postoperative analgesia. Positioning is as for a spinal block.

A Tuohy needle is advanced towards the epidural space, with continuous or intermittent pressure applied to a saline-filled syringe attached to the distal end of the needle. As the ligamentum flavum is breached there is a sudden loss of resistance. An epidural catheter is threaded down the needle, which is then removed and discarded.

Combined spinal epidural

Combined spinal–epidural (CSE) block is when both procedures are performed at the same time, either as a 'needle through needle' technique or as two separate procedures at different vertebral levels. It has the advantage of rapid onset (spinal) and the ability to supplement with the epidural component as the spinal anaesthetic wears off (e.g. postoperative analgesia or prolonged surgery).

The injected drugs act directly on the spinal cord and nerve roots, blocking sensory, motor and autonomic nerve transmission. LA and opiates given together have a synergistic effect.

Nerve plexus blockade

The two main ways of locating the targeted nerve are to use a nerve stimulator or ultrasound. Either technique can be used or both together.

Although rare, inadvertent intravenous injection of LA and/or LA toxicity are recognized complications. Full resuscitation facilities, including drugs and equipment to perform tracheal intubation, must be available whenever a nerve block is performed.

Repeated syringe aspiration on injecting LA is important to prevent inadvertent intravenous injection.

Nerve damage is rare but the issue should be discussed with the patient.

Nerve stimulator The needle is attached to a variable electrical current. It is initially set to 1–2 mA with a frequency of 1–2 Hz. As the nerve is approached, a motor response in the muscles supplied by the nerve is elicited. The current is reduced as the nerve is approached, aiming to produce the best motor response at the lowest current. When the correct needle position is achieved, muscle twitch will usually disappear at a current of 0.2–0.3 mA (threshold). If twitches persist down to a very low amperage, it suggests intraneural placement and the needle should be resited. The injection should be pain free – if pain does occur, the injection must be stopped and the needle repositioned. Twitches disappear as the LA is injected, due to the conductive properties of the LA.

Ultrasound (Figure 22.2) Advantages are direct vision of the needle's entire length and tip throughout all stages of needle advancement as well as seeing the spread of LA as it is given. Other potential advantages include:
- higher success rate;
- quicker to perform;
- quicker onset of block;
- smaller doses of anaesthetic used;
- less pain in performing;
- increased patient satisfaction.

Some common nerve blocks

- **Interscalene block** provides surgical anaesthesia to shoulder, upper arm and forearm. The upper, middle and lower trunks of the brachial plexus are blocked as they lie in the interscalene groove (between the scalenus anterior and scalenus medius), within a fascial sheath. The groove is located at the level of C6 (corresponding to the cricoid cartilage) at the lateral border of the sternocleidomastoid.
- **Axillary block** is used for surgery of the elbow, forearm and hand. It blocks the radial (C5–T1), ulnar (C7–T1), median (C6–T1) and musculocutaneous (C5–7) nerves high in the axilla, lateral to the pectoralis minor. The nerves lie within a fascial sheath with the axillary artery and vein (the latter is not always within the sheath).
- **Femoral nerve block** is used for surgery of the anterior thigh, knee and quadriceps tendon. The femoral nerve (L2–4) is the largest branch arising from the lumbar plexus. It is located lateral to the femoral artery, in the inguinal crease, just distal to the inguinal ligament. Stimulation of quadriceps (patella twitch) indicates correct needle placement. If used in combination with a sciatic nerve block, total anaesthesia distal to the mid thigh is produced.
- **Popliteal block** affects the sciatic nerve (L4–S3) proximal to its bifurcation into the common peroneal nerve (L4–S2) and the tibial nerve (L4–S3). It provides anaesthesia below the knee, excluding that supplied by the saphenous nerve (a terminal branch of the femoral nerve). The injection is at the apex of a triangle where the popliteal crease is the base and the sides are composed of the tendons of biceps femoris (lateral) and semitendinosus and semimembranosus (medial).

Figure 23.1 Aspiration

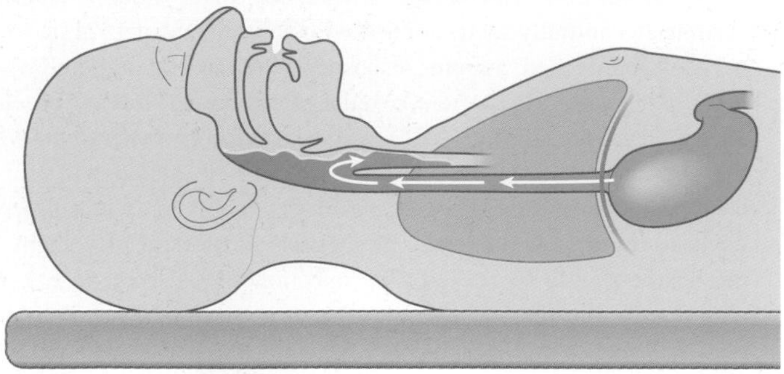

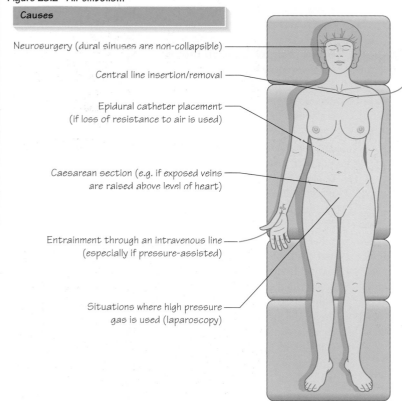

Regurgitation of gastric contents can happen in any patient who does not have fully functioning upper airway protective reflexes Those at risk include:

- Inadequate period of preoperative starvation
- Delayed gastric emptying (e.g. opiates, pain, bowel obstruction, pregnancy at term; see Figure 6.2)
- Insufficient/lack of cricoid pressure at induction of anaesthesia early extubation in an at-risk patient

Treatment

- 100% oxygen
- Call for help
- 30% Head-down position to prevent/limit aspiration
- Oropharyngeal suction
- Tracheal intubation if needed, including tracheal suctioning
- Postoperatively: physiotherapy, oxygen. Some advocate antibiotics and steroids

Signs

- Gastric contents visible within breathing circuit/airway adjunct (e.g. LMA)
- $\downarrow S_aO_2$
- Wheeze/stridor
- Tachycardia
- $\uparrow$Airway pressure

Figure 23.2 Air embolism

Causes

Neurosurgery (dural sinuses are non-collapsible)

Central line insertion/removal

Epidural catheter placement (if loss of resistance to air is used)

Caesarean section (e.g. if exposed veins are raised above level of heart)

Entrainment through an intravenous line (especially if pressure-assisted)

Situations where high pressure gas is used (laparoscopy)

Signs

- $\uparrow$HR
- $\downarrow$BP
- $\downarrow S_aO_2$
- $\downarrow$ETCO$_2$ (acute due to ventilation–perfusion mismatch)
- Murmur (millwheel, due to air circulating around the cardiac chambers)

Treatment

- 100% Oxygen
- Airway, breathing, circulation and call for help
- Flood surgical site with saline
- Position patient in Trendelenburg/left lateral decubitus position
- Consider inserting a central venous catheter to aspirate gas
- Consider hyperbaric chamber if indicated

Emergencies are not common but when they do occur they are often life threatening and require immediate action. They are often unforeseen and may have a non-specific presentation. Moreover, many need prompt diagnosis and treatment if disaster is to be averted. Some disasters happen 'out of the blue' but some occur or are recognized late due to other factors, such as distraction, tiredness, work and time pressures, poor communication, etc.

Factors in the mnemonic **COVER ABCD** accounts for approximately 95% of critical incidents. It is an example of an algorithm that can be used as an *aide-mémoire* to work through during an acute event. Always ensure senior help is sought early.

Anaesthesia at a Glance, First Edition. Julian Stone and William Fawcett.

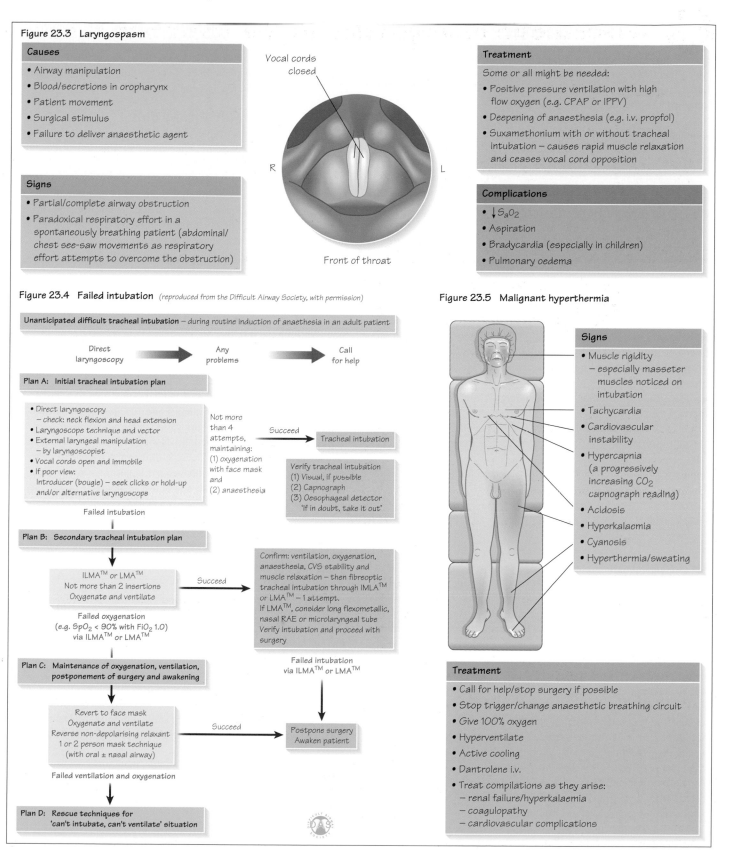

Figure 23.3 Laryngospasm

Causes

- Airway manipulation
- Blood/secretions in oropharynx
- Patient movement
- Surgical stimulus
- Failure to deliver anaesthetic agent

Signs

- Partial/complete airway obstruction
- Paradoxical respiratory effort in a spontaneously breathing patient (abdominal/chest see-saw movements as respiratory effort attempts to overcome the obstruction)

Vocal cords closed

R L

Front of throat

Treatment

Some or all might be needed:

- Positive pressure ventilation with high flow oxygen (e.g. CPAP or IPPV)
- Deepening of anaesthesia (e.g. i.v. propfol)
- Suxamethonium with or without tracheal intubation – causes rapid muscle relaxation and ceases vocal cord opposition

Complications

- $\downarrow S_aO_2$
- Aspiration
- Bradycardia (especially in children)
- Pulmonary oedema

Figure 23.4 Failed intubation *(reproduced from the Difficult Airway Society, with permission)*

Unanticipated difficult tracheal intubation – during routine induction of anaesthesia in an adult patient

Direct laryngoscopy → Any problems → Call for help

Plan A: Initial tracheal intubation plan

- Direct laryngoscopy
  – check: neck flexion and head extension
- Laryngoscope technique and vector
- External laryngeal manipulation
  – by laryngoscopist
- Vocal cords open and immobile
- If poor view:
  Introducer (bougie) – seek clicks or hold-up and/or alternative laryngoscope

Not more than 4 attempts, maintaining:
(1) oxygenation with face mask and
(2) anaesthesia

→ Succeed → Tracheal intubation

Verify tracheal intubation
(1) Visual, if possible
(2) Capnograph
(3) Oesophageal detector
'If in doubt, take it out'

Failed intubation

Plan B: Secondary tracheal intubation plan

ILMA™ or LMA™
Not more than 2 insertions
Oxygenate and ventilate

→ Succeed →

Confirm: ventilation, oxygenation, anaesthesia, CVS stability and muscle relaxation – then fibreoptic tracheal intubation through IMLA™ or LMA™ – 1 attempt.
If LMA™, consider long flexometallic, nasal RAE or microlaryngeal tube
Verify intubation and proceed with surgery

Failed oxygenation
(e.g. SpO_2 < 90% with FiO_2 1.0)
via ILMA™ or LMA™

Failed intubation
via ILMA™ or LMA™

Plan C: Maintenance of oxygenation, ventilation, postponement of surgery and awakening

Revert to face mask
Oxygenate and ventilate
Reverse non-depolarising relaxant
1 or 2 person mask technique
(with oral ± nasal airway)

→ Succeed →

Postpone surgery
Awaken patient

Failed ventilation and oxygenation

Plan D: Rescue techniques for 'can't intubate, can't ventilate' situation

Figure 23.5 Malignant hyperthermia

Signs

- Muscle rigidity
  – especially masseter muscles noticed on intubation
- Tachycardia
- Cardiovascular instability
- Hypercapnia
  (a progressively increasing CO_2 capnograph reading)
- Acidosis
- Hyperkalaemia
- Cyanosis
- Hyperthermia/sweating

Treatment

- Call for help/stop surgery if possible
- Stop trigger/change anaesthetic breathing circuit
- Give 100% oxygen
- Hyperventilate
- Active cooling
- Dantrolene i.v.
- Treat compilations as they arise:
  – renal failure/hyperkalaemia
  – coagulopathy
  – cardiovascular complications

Colour – saturation, central cyanosis;

Oxygen – ensure adequate and correct delivery;

Ventilation – e.g. breathing circuit, air entry, CO_2 trace, vaporizer;

Endotracheal tube – kinks, obstruction, endobronchial;

Review monitors – correctly sited, checked, calibrated;

Airway – failed intubation, laryngeal spasm, foreign body, aspiration;

Breathing – difficult to ventilate, e.g. tube occlusion, bronchospasm, pneumothorax, aspiration, lack of neuromuscular blocking drug (NMBD), pulmonary oedema;

Circulation – hypotension: excess anaesthetic agent, dysrhythmia, myocardial ischaemia/MI, hypovolaemia from any cause (e.g. dehydration, bleeding), sepsis, tension pneumothorax, sympathetic block (e.g. spinal or epidural anaesthetic);

Drugs – anaphylaxis, wrong drug/dose/route;

Embolism – air/fat/cement/amniotic fluid;

Others – related to CVP line (pneumothorax [see Chapter 25]/cardiac tamponade); awareness; endocrine and metabolic (MH, phaeochromocytoma).

Aspiration

Inhalation of gastric contents can occur in patients who do not have fully functional upper airway reflexes (Figure 23.1). Impaired protective airway reflexes can be due to:
- a reduced conscious level from any cause;
- neuromuscular blocking agents;
- central nervous system disorders, e.g. stroke, bulbar palsy.

General anaesthesia obtunds airway reflexes that normally function to protect the respiratory tract from soiling by regurgitated vomitus. Patients for elective surgery are starved for a minimum of 6 hours to minimize the risk of this happening. Regurgitation can occur in any patient but this is a particular risk when surgery needs to proceed before 6 hours of nil by mouth (e.g. trauma, vascular injury) and in patients who might have residual gastric contents despite delay (e.g. bowel obstruction, acute pain, opiate administration, pregnant women at term).

Causes of reduced level of consciousness include:
- head injury;
- drugs, general anaesthesia;
- opiates;
- sedatives, e.g. benzodiazepines;
- alcohol;
- intracranial pathology, e.g. cerebrovascular accident;
- metabolic, e.g. diabetic coma.

Air embolism

Air embolism results from inadvertent introduction of air into the circulation, usually via the venous system (Figure 23.2). Air bubbles pass into the right atrium and ventricle, where they can cause a reduction in right ventricular cardiac output because the non-compressible blood becomes frothy as it is mixed with compressible gas. Bubbles can then pass into the pulmonary circulation, causing ventilation–perfusion mismatch and hypoxia. Paradoxical emboli can occur via cardiac septal defects, resulting in coronary and cerebral emboli.

As well as supportive treatment, which aims to maintain cardiovascular and respiratory function, specific measures include repositioning the patient to limit the harm that the air emboli might cause. By placing the patient on their left side (left lateral decubitus position) and tilting the head end of the operating table down and the foot end up (Trendelenburg), emboli should remain in the apex of the right ventricle and not enter the pulmonary circulation. A central venous catheter can then be introduced and the gas aspirated. If nitrous oxide is being used it must be discontinued as it will increase the size of emboli.

Fat embolism and bone cement implantation syndrome are discussed in Chapter 26.

Laryngospasm

Laryngospasm is the complete or partial adduction of the vocal cords, resulting in a variable degree of airway obstruction (Figure 23.3). The extent of desaturation depends on the length of time of obstruction, if preoxygenation occurred, the age of the patient (more rapid in children who have higher O_2 consumption), as well as pre-existing lung pathology (e.g. COPD). It is more likely to occur at lighter planes of anaesthesia, that is at induction and emergence.

Failed or difficult intubation

This is when a patient's trachea cannot be intubated or it proves unexpectedly difficult to perform. The causes of this are discussed in Chapter 16.

The algorithm shown in Figure 23.4 should be followed. Before induction of anaesthesia, plans should always be in place in case the initial course fails. Sequential steps should be taken to improve the chance of successful intubation. Delay in progressing to the next step must be avoided in order to avoid hypoxaemia.

Patients come to harm from failure to oxygenate, not failure to intubate.

Simple steps that should be taken to improve the view of the larynx at laryngoscopy include:
- ensuring optimum patient position, i.e. neck flexion and head extension ('sniffing the morning air');
- external laryngeal manipulation;
- use of a different laryngoscope blade (e.g. a long blade in larger patients).

Although rare, the situation of neither being able to ventilate nor intubate (CICV – see also Chapters 4 and 16) must be recognized and treated with either needle or surgical cricothyroidotomy.

In a rapid sequence induction, if simple steps to aid intubation (Figure 23.4 Plan A) are not successful then the patient is woken up and surgery postponed. If postponement is not possible, as in a life-threatening condition, then an alternative technique is used such as LMA or ProSeal LMA (Intravent, Bucks UK).

Malignant hyperthermia (MH)

This occurs after exposure to a triggering agent (volatile anaesthetics or suxamethonium) and results in loss of normal calcium homeostasis within skeletal muscle cells (Figure 23.5). The incidence is 1/5000–20 000. The genetic defect is thought to be the ryanodine receptor, coded for by a gene on Chromosome 19 and autosomal dominant in inheritance. Hypermetabolism leads to hypoxia, hypercapnia, hyperthermia and acidosis. Cell damage results in release of potassium, myoglobin and creatine kinase.

The treatment of MH includes removal of the triggering agent, 100% oxygen, active cooling measures (e.g. stop any active warming, ice packs around head, neck and in axillae, etc., tepid sponging, bladder irrigation with cold water) and dantrolene i.v. Dantrolene is a skeletal muscle relaxant, which inhibits calcium release from the sarcoplasmic reticulum. It is given at a dose of 1 mg/kg and can be repeated up to 10 mg/kg. Once stable, the patient is transferred to intensive care. The mortality from MH has been reduced from 80% to <5% since the introduction of dantrolene.

All patients with suspected MH should be referred for investigation; a muscle biopsy is taken and the tissue exposed to caffeine and halothane (contracture test). Muscle contraction is a positive result and patients are divided into positive, negative and equivocal groups based on this result. MH-positive and equivocal patients need to wear a 'medic alert' bracelet and must receive an MH-safe anaesthetic for subsequent operations (e.g. a regional technique or total intravenous anaesthesia).

Figure 24.1   Anaphylaxis

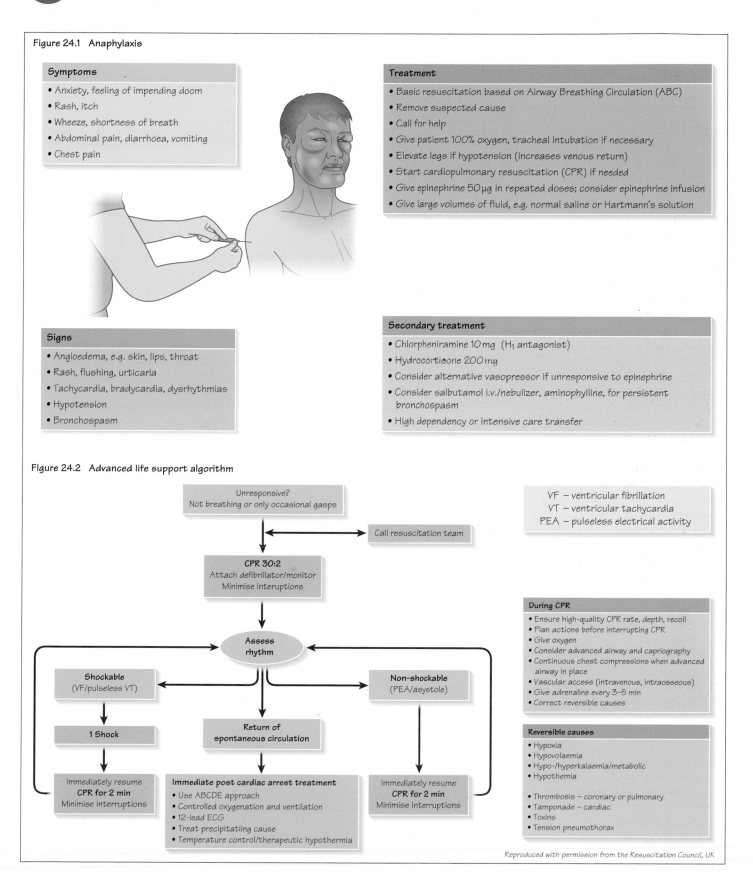

Symptoms

- Anxiety, feeling of impending doom
- Rash, itch
- Wheeze, shortness of breath
- Abdominal pain, diarrhoea, vomiting
- Chest pain

Treatment

- Basic resuscitation based on Airway Breathing Circulation (ABC)
- Remove suspected cause
- Call for help
- Give patient 100% oxygen, tracheal intubation if necessary
- Elevate legs if hypotension (increases venous return)
- Start cardiopulmonary resuscitation (CPR) if needed
- Give epinephrine 50 µg in repeated doses; consider epinephrine infusion
- Give large volumes of fluid, e.g. normal saline or Hartmann's solution

Signs

- Angioedema, e.g. skin, lips, throat
- Rash, flushing, urticaria
- Tachycardia, bradycardia, dysrhythmias
- Hypotension
- Bronchospasm

Secondary treatment

- Chlorpheniramine 10 mg (H_1 antagonist)
- Hydrocortisone 200 mg
- Consider alternative vasopressor if unresponsive to epinephrine
- Consider salbutamol i.v./nebulizer, aminophylline, for persistent bronchospasm
- High dependency or intensive care transfer

Figure 24.2   Advanced life support algorithm

Unresponsive?
Not breathing or only occasional gasps

Call resuscitation team

VF – ventricular fibrillation
VT – ventricular tachycardia
PEA – pulseless electrical activity

CPR 30:2
Attach defibrillator/monitor
Minimise interuptions

Assess rhythm

Shockable
(VF/pulseless VT)

Non-shockable
(PEA/asystole)

1 Shock

Return of
spontaneous circulation

Immediately resume
CPR for 2 min
Minimise interruptions

Immediate post cardiac arrest treatment
- Use ABCDE approach
- Controlled oxygenation and ventilation
- 12-lead ECG
- Treat precipitatiing cause
- Temperature control/therapeutic hypothermia

Immediately resume
CPR for 2 min
Minimise interruptions

During CPR

- Ensure high-quality CPR rate, depth, recoil
- Plan actions before interrupting CPR
- Give oxygen
- Consider advanced airway and capriography
- Continuous chest compressions when advanced airway in place
- Vascular access (intravenous, intraosseous)
- Give adrenaline every 3–5 min
- Correct reversible causes

Reversible causes

- Hypoxia
- Hypovolaemia
- Hypo-/hyperkalaemia/metabolic
- Hypothemia

- Thrombosis – coronary or pulmonary
- Tamponade – cardiac
- Toxins
- Tension pneumothorax

Reproduced with permission from the Resuscitation Council, UK

Anaesthesia at a Glance, First Edition. Julian Stone and William Fawcett.
© 2013 Julian Stone and William Fawcett. Published 2013 by John Wiley & Sons, Ltd.   **59**

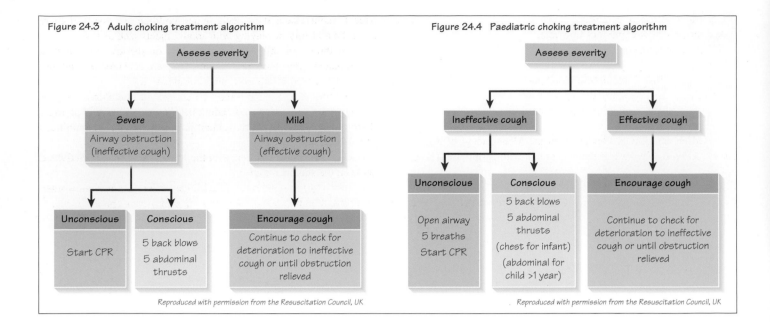

Figure 24.3 Adult choking treatment algorithm

Assess severity

Severe
Airway obstruction
(ineffective cough)

Mild
Airway obstruction
(effective cough)

Unconscious
Start CPR

Conscious
5 back blows
5 abdominal
thrusts

Encourage cough
Continue to check for
deterioration to ineffective
cough or until obstruction
relieved

Reproduced with permission from the Resuscitation Council, UK

Figure 24.4 Paediatric choking treatment algorithm

Assess severity

Ineffective cough

Effective cough

Unconscious
Open airway
5 breaths
Start CPR

Conscious
5 back blows
5 abdominal
thrusts
(chest for infant)
(abdominal for
child >1 year)

Encourage cough
Continue to check for
deterioration to ineffective
cough or until obstruction
relieved

Reproduced with permission from the Resuscitation Council, UK

Anaphylaxis

This is an acute severe type 1 hypersensitivity reaction when an antigen (trigger) reacts with immunoglobulin IgE bound to histamine-rich mast cells and basophils. The clinical features are some or all of: oedema, rash, wheeze, shortness of breath and circulatory collapse (Figure 24.1). The incidence during anaesthesia is approximately 1/10 000–1/20 000. On allergen exposure (after previous exposure which will have sensitized the patient) there is a large IgE-mediated release of histamine, complement and other inflammatory mediators. Within anaesthesia the commonest causative agents are neuromuscular blocking agents (60%), latex (20%) and antibiotics (15%). Most reactions occur soon after administration but can be delayed by up to an hour. Although intravenous drugs are the commonest cause in anaesthesia, skin cleaning preparations (e.g. iodine or chlorhexidine) are also well-recognized causes.

Follow-up and investigation of suspected anaphylaxis is important. It should also be considered in unexpected perioperative critical incidents (e.g. unexplained perioperative cardiac arrest, unexplained hypotension or bronchospasm, widespread rash, angioedema).

Three blood samples should be taken for mast cell tryptase:

1 as soon as possible (but without interfering with treatment or resuscitation);

2 1–2 hours later;

3 24 hours later or at follow-up.

Later investigation includes referral to an allergy specialist, skin prick testing and intradermal testing (more sensitive but less specific). Specific IgE can be detected by using a method involving fluorescence labelling and the allergen (or drug) bound to a solid sponge-like matrix. Assays exist for specific IgE (e.g. against succinylcholine, other neuromuscular blocking agents and commonly used antibiotics). When an allergy is known, the patient must wear an allergy bracelet at all times whilst an inpatient.

Cardiac arrest

Anaesthetists are part of the in-hospital cardiac arrest team. Basic life support should be performed until advanced life support can be instituted (Figure 24.2). Chest compressions should be to a depth of 5–6 cm and at a rate of 100–120 per minute. Only someone appropriately skilled should perform tracheal intubation and it must cause minimal interruption to chest compressions. Current practice emphasizes 'the importance of minimally-interrupted high-quality chest compressions throughout any ALS intervention' (e.g. intubation, defibrillation) (Resuscitation Council, UK).

After successful resuscitation, intensive care treatment will pay particular attention to establishing normal oxygen and CO_2 levels, coronary artery patency, seizure control, normal blood sugar and therapeutic hypothermia.

Status asthmaticus

This is a severe acute exacerbation of asthma refractory to conventional β2 agonist therapy and is a medical emergency. The signs are:

• tachypnoea;

• use of accessory respiratory muscles (e.g. abdominal, sternocleidomastoid), and intercostal and subcostal recession;

• wheeze might be minimal or absent;

• tachycardia;

• pulsus paradoxus >10 mmHg (a reduction in blood pressure on inspiration);

• sweating;

• tiring;

• confusion.

Treatment consists of:

• give supplemental oxygen to maintain S_aO_2 94–98%;

• β2 agonist (either salbutamol or terbutaline) via O_2 driven nebulizer;

• continuous nebulization can be used if there is a poor initial response;

• intravenous β2 agonists should only be used when the inhaled route is unreliable;

• steroids – either oral prednisolone or i.v. hydrocortisone;

• nebulized ipratropium (anticholinergic);

• consider i.v. magnesium sulphate when life-threatening or poor initial response to treatment; aminophylline might also be considered in this situation.

Referral to intensive care if:

- deteriorating peak expiratory flow rate;
- persisting or worsening hypoxia;
- hypercapnia;
- falling pH/rising H^+ on arterial blood gas;
- exhaustion, feeble respiration;
- drowsiness, confusion, altered conscious state;
- respiratory arrest.

(Based on BTS/SIGN Guideline on the Management of Asthma, 2009 (section 6.3) www.brit-thoracic.org.uk with permission.)

Choking/airway obstruction

Everyone involved in patient care should be able to recognize and treat choking (Figures 24.3 and 24.4). It might occur whilst eating, and the patient might clutch their neck. When children are involved there might be a history of playing with small objects such as toys.

Chest thrusts in children are performed on the lower sternum, a fingerbreadth above the xiphisternum. They are delivered in a sharper way and at a slower rate than chest compressions.

Abdominal thrusts should only be performed in children >1 year old. They are performed by standing behind the child and applying a sharp upward and inward movement halfway between the umbilicus and xiphisternum.

Back blows are carried out with the flat of the hand, and delivered between the shoulder blades.

Do not perform blind or repeated finger sweeps as this can worsen the obstruction by pushing objects further into the respiratory tree.

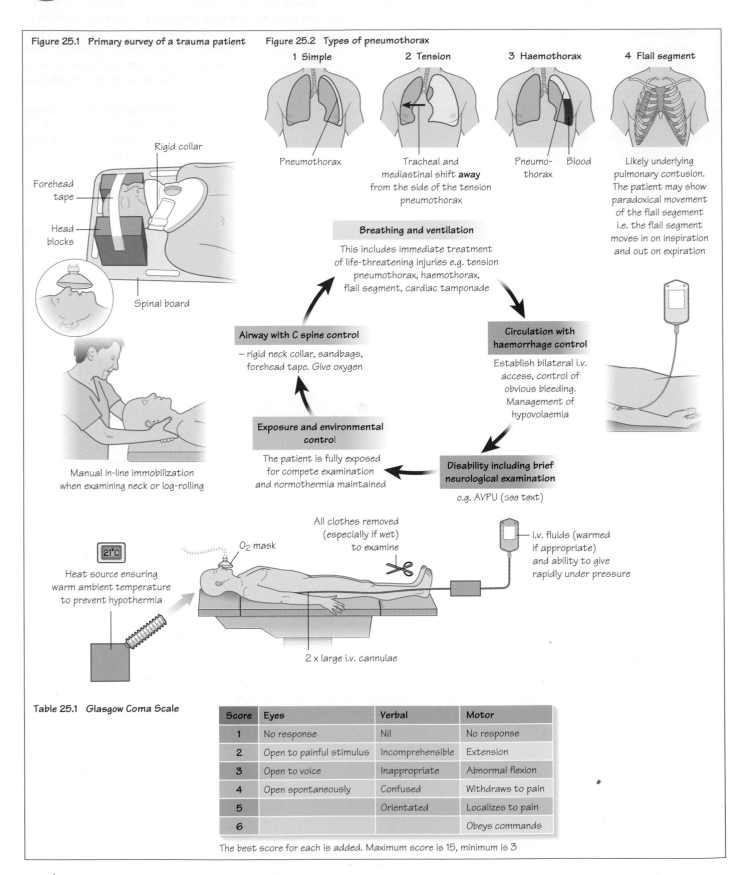

Figure 25.1 Primary survey of a trauma patient

Rigid collar

Forehead tape

Head blocks

Spinal board

Manual in-line immobilization when examining neck or log-rolling

Figure 25.2 Types of pneumothorax

1 Simple — Pneumothorax

2 Tension — Tracheal and mediastinal shift **away** from the side of the tension pneumothorax

3 Haemothorax — Pneumothorax, Blood

4 Flail segment — Likely underlying pulmonary contusion. The patient may show paradoxical movement of the flail segement i.e. the flail segment moves in on inspiration and out on expiration

Breathing and ventilation

This includes immediate treatment of life-threatening injuries e.g. tension pneumothorax, haemothorax, flail segment, cardiac tamponade

Airway with C spine control

– rigid neck collar, sandbags, forehead tape. Give oxygen

Circulation with haemorrhage control

Establish bilateral i.v. access, control of obvious bleeding. Management of hypovolaemia

Exposure and environmental control

The patient is fully exposed for compete examination and normothermia maintained

Disability including brief neurological examination

e.g. AVPU (see text)

Heat source ensuring warm ambient temperature to prevent hypothermia

21°C

O_2 mask

All clothes removed (especially if wet) to examine

2 x large i.v. cannulae

i.v. fluids (warmed if appropriate) and ability to give rapidly under pressure

Table 25.1 Glasgow Coma Scale

Score	Eyes	Verbal	Motor
1	No response	Nil	No response
2	Open to painful stimulus	Incomprehensible	Extension
3	Open to voice	Inappropriate	Abnormal flexion
4	Open spontaneously	Confused	Withdraws to pain
5		Orientated	Localizes to pain
6			Obeys commands

The best score for each is added. Maximum score is 15, minimum is 3

Anaesthesia at a Glance, First Edition. Julian Stone and William Fawcett.

All patients with significant trauma should undergo standardized trauma treatment. In the UK, this is based on the Advanced Trauma Life Support (ATLS) protocol. This consists of a primary survey, in which resuscitation and identification and treatment of life-threatening injuries occurs, followed by a secondary survey, consisting of a complete head-to-toe assessment. This is followed by definitive treatment of injuries.

Primary survey

Airway plus cervical spine control High-flow oxygen is given via a facemask. If the patient has a reduced level of consciousness, or is at risk of regurgitation, an endotracheal tube is passed into the trachea. In significant trauma, bony cervical spine injury is assumed until it can be excluded by imaging and examination. In all cases before cervical spine injury is excluded, manual in-line stabilization must be used to limit neck movement when a rigid neck collar and head blocks are not being used.

Breathing plus ventilation Chest injuries are identified and treated (Figure 25.1). Mechanical ventilation might be needed to avoid hypoxia and hypercapnia, especially in patients with a head injury.

Circulation with haemorrhage control Two large-bore cannulae are inserted and fluid resuscitation commenced. Blood is given if the haematocrit is <30% or haemoglobin <10g/dL. All fluids should be warmed to limit hypothermia and potential coagulopathy. Direct pressure is applied to obvious bleeding sources. Fluids might need to be given through a rapid infusion device under pressure in order to speed delivery.

Causes of hypotension These include:
- hypovolaemia
- cardiac contusion or tamponade
- aortic rupture
- neurogenic shock
- tension pneumothorax.

Disability This is recorded using the AVPU scale (Alert, responds to a Verbal stimulus, responds to a Painful stimulus, Unresponsive) or the Glasgow Coma Score (GCS). AVPU is a brief and rapid way of assessing level of consciousness; GCS is a more detailed method, giving a score between 3 and 15 (Table 25.1).

Environment/exposure The patient is fully undressed and attention paid to maintaining normothermia and keeping dry.

Multiple trauma The anaesthetist plays a pivotal role in the treatment of the patient with multiple trauma, often acting as the team leader and liaising between specialties (e.g. radiology, surgery, orthopaedics). For these patients, special attention should be paid to:
- oxygenation and airway management (airway, breathing and circulation – ABC);
- analgesia.

Secondary survey

A history is taken, which should ask as a minimum (mnemonic = AMPLE):
- allergies;
- medications;

- previous medical history;
- last oral intake;
- events immediately before injury.

Details from other people are important as the patient might be incapable of providing accurate information due to reduced conscious level, endotracheal tube *in situ* or intoxication (e.g. drugs or alcohol). The mechanism of injury, as well as the degree of force involved, should also be sought (e.g. thrown from a car, not wearing a seat belt, distance fallen, etc.).

Gastric stasis will occur due to pain and trauma and it is important to recognize that most patients will be at aspiration risk if they have a reduced level of consciousness or need an anaesthetic. If a gastric tube is needed, it should be passed orally rather than nasally in case there is a basal skull fracture.

A thorough examination is carried out of the entire patient from head-to-toe, both front and back.

Head This includes looking for lacerations, haematomas, orbit and eye injuries, and mid-face injuries. The signs of a **basal skull fracture** are:
- raccoon eyes;
- mastoid bruising (Battle's sign);
- subhyaloid haemorrhage;
- haemotympanum;
- CSF rhinorrhoea/otorrhoea.

Chest Life-threatening chest injuries are identified and treated (as in the primary survey).

Abdomen Intra-abdominal bleeding should be considered if hypotension persists despite fluid resuscitation. Pain, distension and bruising are noted. Examination of the external genitalia might reveal bleeding from the urethral meatus; rectal examination should be performed to assess anal sphincter tone (reduced in spinal injury) and prostate position (e.g. urethral injury). Urine output is monitored after catheterization.

Long bones Fractures contribute to blood loss (e.g. a closed femoral fracture can lose 1–2 litres) as well as causing pain. Pain, neurovascular injury, compartment syndrome and rhabdomyolysis should all be considered and treated.

Investigations

These include: full blood count, urea and electrolytes, cross matched blood. If blood needs to be given immediately then O negative should be given whilst a full cross match is performed.

Cervical spine, chest and pelvis X rays are taken as a minimum, plus other injured areas as indicated. Ultrasound as well as CT/MRI imaging are used as required (e.g. intra-abdominal injuries).

Prophylactic antibiotics are given and tetanus toxoid if not covered.

If at any stage the patient deteriorates (e.g. reduction in level of consciousness, hypotension, tachycardia, tachypnoea), a further primary survey is performed in order to identify and treat the cause.

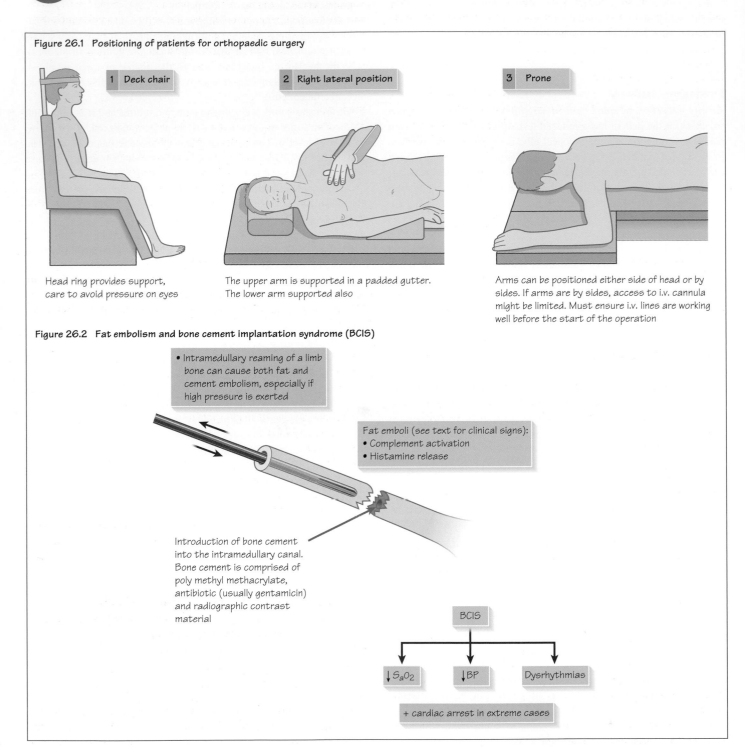

Figure 26.1 Positioning of patients for orthopaedic surgery

1 Deck chair

Head ring provides support, care to avoid pressure on eyes

2 Right lateral position

The upper arm is supported in a padded gutter. The lower arm supported also

3 Prone

Arms can be positioned either side of head or by sides. If arms are by sides, access to i.v. cannula might be limited. Must ensure i.v. lines are working well before the start of the operation

Figure 26.2 Fat embolism and bone cement implantation syndrome (BCIS)

• Intramedullary reaming of a limb bone can cause both fat and cement embolism, especially if high pressure is exerted

Fat emboli (see text for clinical signs):
• Complement activation
• Histamine release

Introduction of bone cement into the intramedullary canal. Bone cement is comprised of poly methyl methacrylate, antibiotic (usually gentamicin) and radiographic contrast material

BCIS

$\downarrow S_aO_2$ | $\downarrow$BP | Dysrhythmias

+ cardiac arrest in extreme cases

Anaesthesia at a Glance, First Edition. Julian Stone and William Fawcett.

Orthopaedic anaesthesia encompasses a range of operations, from minor procedures on young patients (e.g. arthroscopy) to the commonly performed joint replacements (hip and knee, often in elderly patients) and major spinal surgery, including those with unstable fractures. Urgent orthopaedics cases include open fractures and neurovascular deficit.

The anaesthetist must pay particular attention to the following during orthopaedic operations:
- Great care must be taken to ensure that the patient's airway is secure and that the endotracheal tube (ETT) or LMA being used is securely fastened so as to prevent dislodgement, especially when access to the head and neck during the operation might be difficult, e.g. under surgical drapes or when prone.
- Pressure points must be protected to prevent nerve or soft tissue damage. The use of gel pads, as well as padding and supports, helps avoid this.
- Direct pressure on the orbit must be avoided at all times in order to avoid retinal artery thrombosis and visual impairment postoperatively.
- The patient's limbs must not be over stretched (e.g. shoulder) so as to avoid nerve plexus injury (e.g. brachial plexus palsy).
- Do not abduct the upper arm >90 degrees from body as this might cause posterior shoulder displacement.

Preoperative care
Assessment
Early fracture fixation relieves pain and is a reason for taking patients to theatre as soon as is appropriate. Patients need to be fully assessed and often require optimizing before their operation, especially the elderly, with specific attention to:
- fluid resuscitation
- anaemia
- electrolyte imbalances
- normothermia.

Medical conditions
Some musculoskeletal conditions present more commonly for orthopaedic procedures (e.g. rheumatoid arthritis (RA), osteoarthritis and ankylosing spondylitis).

Problems can include:
- Pain: even positioning an awake patient in the anaesthetic room might exacerbate joint symptoms. Pain can markedly limit exercise tolerance.
- Airway and cervical spine: up to 80% of RA patients have neck involvement, including instability and subluxation. Care must be taken when moving the head and neck position as well as transferring patients.
- Temporomandibular joint involvement can reduce mouth opening, hindering intubation or laryngeal mask insertion.
- Extra-articular disease might be present, e.g. restrictive lung disease and cardiac involvement (rare).
- Current medication must be reviewed, e.g. if taking corticosteroids, extra steroid might need to be given in the perioperative period.

The cause of a fall must be established to differentiate between a simple trip, an alcohol or drug-related fall, and those due to cardiovascular or cerebrovascular causes (e.g. postural hypotension, transient ischaemic attack or dysrhythmia).

Peroperative care
Positioning
Surgical access often requires the patient to be positioned in a specific way during the operation, other than just supine; examples include:
- for access to back, spine or heel: prone position (Figure 26.1);
- for access to shoulder: deck chair position (Figure 26.2);
- for access to hip: lateral position (Figure 26.3).

Infection
Strict aseptic conditions must be adhered to during orthopaedic surgery, especially when a prosthesis is introduced (e.g. a new joint in the hip or knee replacement). In these cases antibiotic prophylaxis is given at the start of surgery and continued postoperatively. If a pneumatic tourniquet is used to prevent blood loss intraoperatively, the antibiotics must be given before tourniquet inflation. All staff present must wear surgical masks.

Fat embolism syndrome (FES)
Fat emboli can form as a result of fractures; most commonly from multitrauma of the long bones and pelvis. The diagnosis of FES requires at least one major plus three minor of the following criteria.
- Major criteria:
  - petechiae;
  - hypoxaemia;
  - pulmonary oedema.
- Minor criteria:
  - tachycardia >110 beats per min;
  - pyrexia >38.5°C;
  - visible emboli on fundoscopy;
  - urinary fat;
  - fat globules in sputum;
  - elevated ESR;
  - sudden fall in platelets or haematocrit.

Treatment is supportive, particularly for cardiovascular and respiratory systems. Prevention is important, and early treatment of fractures might reduce the incidence. Mortality can be 10–20%.

Bone cement implantation syndrome (BCIS)
Orthopaedic bone cement is often used during joint (e.g. hip) arthroplasty. BCIS is characterized by some or all of:
- hypoxia
- hypotension
- cardiac dysrhythmias
- cardiac arrest.

The cause is not fully understood but is likely to be multifactorial, including fat emboli, medullary reaming (which produces high intramedullary pressure), complement activation and histamine release (Figure 26.4).

To reduce the incidence, higher-risk patients should be identified (e.g. those with cardiovascular, respiratory or metastatic disease) and the use of invasive BP monitoring should be considered in these patients. Preventive measures include adequate fluid balance during the operation and increased inspired O_2 concentration during cement insertion. Use of a non-cemented technique in those at increased risk should be considered.

Regional and central blocks

Operations involving the pelvis and lower limbs lend themselves well to central neuraxial blockade (either spinal or epidural analgesia). The patient can receive sedation during the operation, with the potential for more rapid recovery in the immediate postoperative period.

Many limb operations are well suited to a regional anaesthetic block (see Chapter 22).

In both techniques the patient can remain awake throughout the operation or receive sedation. In certain groups of patients it avoids the potential complications of general anaesthesia, such as patients with:

- a difficult airway;
- respiratory disease, e.g. chronic obstructive pulmonary disease, chest infection;
- obesity (blocks may be technically more difficult to perform, see Chapter 27);
- oesophageal reflux.

Tourniquets

These are used after limb exsanguination (either by elevation or use of a compression bandage) to reduce blood loss and to create a bloodless surgical field. Important points when these are used include:

- Avoid other tissue getting caught under the tourniquet, e.g. scrotum.
- The maximum time inflated is 90–120 min (ischaemic time).
- Use is contraindicated in sickle cell disease (including sickle cell trait).
- Special attention is required when the cuff is deflated due to the release into the systemic circulation of ischaemic metabolites, e.g. potassium, lactate, and H^+. This can cause dysrhythmias and hypotension.

Postoperative care
Pain

Options for postoperative analgesia include:

- ongoing analgesia provided by a regional anaesthetic block;
- longer-acting opiates used in spinal anaesthesia, e.g. diamorphine;
- epidural analgesia;
- patient-controlled analgesia (usually morphine) as well as regular paracetamol/anti-inflammatory drugs and weak opiates, e.g. codeine.

Thromboprophylaxis

All immobile patients are at increased risk of thromboembolism – remember Virchow's triad in explaining thrombosis: a change in *vessel wall, flow* or *blood composition* can lead to clot formation.

In the perioperative period patients are at increased risk of deep vein thrombosis and pulmonary embolism due to immobility and being in a procoagulant state (e.g. dehydration and the stress response). Pelvic and lower limb surgery confer added risk. Patients at risk wear compression stockings (+/− pneumatic compression boots interoperatively), often for several weeks postoperatively.

Patients who do not mobilize after their operation need subcutaneous heparin injections as prophylaxis against thrombus formation. This is most commonly low-molecular-weight heparin. Heparin acts by activating antithrombin III, which itself inhibits thrombin and factor Xa. It is given once daily until mobility returns. Some patients might need to take oral factor Xa inhibitors for several weeks after joint replacement.

Note that at least 12 hours must have elapsed since the last injection of heparin before a spinal anaesthetic can be given due to the increased risk of spinal haematoma and possible subsequent spinal cord compression if bleeding were to occur.

Figure 27.1 Fat distribution patterns

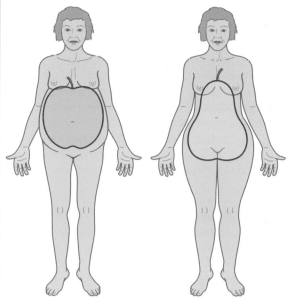

Android obesity   Gynaecoid obesity

Figure 27.2 Complications of obesity

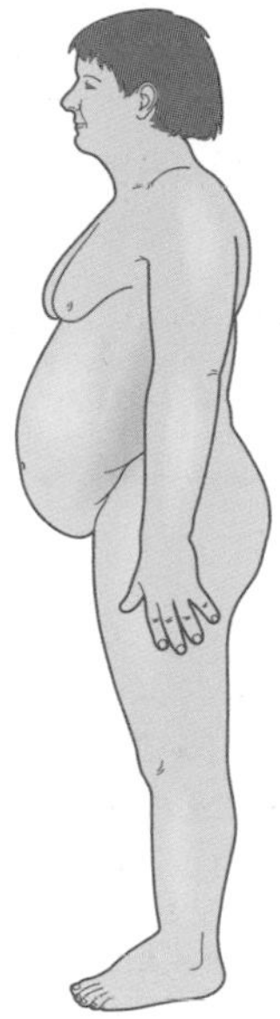

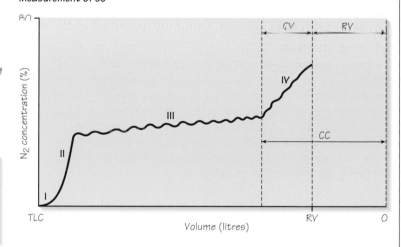

Endocrine
- Diabetes mellitus
- Cushing syndrome
- Hypothyroidism
- Subfertility

Gastrointestinal
- Hiatus hernia
- Gallbladder disease
- Inguinal hernia

Carcinoma
- Breast
- Prostate
- Colorectal
- Endometrial

Musculoskeletal
- Osteoarthritis
- Back pain

CVS disease
- Sudden death
- Cardiomyopathy
- High blood pressure
- Ischaemic heart disease
- Hyperlipidaemia
- Cerebrovascular accident
- Peripheral vascular disease
- Deep venous thrombosis/
  pulmonary embolism
- Cor pulmonale

Respiratory system
- Restrictive lung disease
- Obstructive sleep apnoea
- Obesity hypoventilation syndrome
- Difficult intubation

Genitourinary
- Menstrual problems
- Female incontinence
- Renal calculi

Figure 27.3 Closing capacity (CC) and functional residual capacity (FRC)

When the lung deflates, airway closure will eventually occur: CC is when airway closure can first be detected. CC is normally less than FRC. With increasing age, CC begins to exceed FRC so that above age 40 CC is >FRC when supine and by 60 years old CC is >FRC when standing. In obesity, CC exceeds FRC to a significant degree when supine, independent of age. When CC exceeds FRC, air trapping and airway collapse occur, leading to hypoxaemia.

Patient takes a vital capacity breath of 100%, which goes preferentially to the lung bases. During progressive exhalation into a nitrogen analyser, CC is the point at which basal airway closure starts, leaving a slightly oxygen poor (nitrogen rich) gas exhaled.

> **TLC** – Total lung capacity
> **Phase I** – Anatomic deadspace – pure oxygen
> **Phase II** – Bronchial and alveolar gas
> **Phase III** – Alveolar gas
> **Phase IV** – Sharp rise in nitrogen exhaled, due to airway closure (and hence inspired 100% oxygen did not reach here)

Measurement of CC

Obesity (*obesus* (Latin) = fattened by eating) is a major health problem. Virtually unheard of at the end of the Second World War, it is now a national epidemic. Although multifactorial, a diet high in fat and refined sugars, combined with low levels of activity, have contributed to its increase. Less common causes include endocrine disorders (e.g. Cushing disease and hypothyroidism). There is also a genetic component; adoption studies have shown a 70% chance of obesity if both parents are obese compared to 20% in those of normal weight.

In 2010, 26% of adults (>16 years old) in the UK were classified as obese and 30% of children (2–15 years) were overweight or obese.

Assessing weight and obesity

Body mass index (BMI) is calculated as: weight in kg/height in m^2

BMI <20: underweight
BMI 20–25: normal
BMI 25–30: overweight
BMI 30–35: obese
BMI >35: morbidly obese
BMI >45: super morbidly obese

Ideal body weight in kg (IBW) is calculated as: height in cm −100 for men; height in cm −105 for women.

Although useful as a guide, neither takes account of age, muscle mass or fat distribution. Body fat content for men is 18–25% and for women is 20–30%. A professional footballer would have 12% body fat and a marathon runner 7%.

Fat distribution

Centripetal (android) obesity (Figure 27.1) confers added risk of developing ischaemic heart disease, glucose intolerance, Type 2 diabetes, dyslipidaemias, CVS disease, LV dysfunction and CVA. This is possibly due to products of visceral fat delivered directly to the portal circulation.

In peripheral (gynaecoid) obesity (Figure 27.1) fat accumulates on hips, buttocks and thighs. This is more common in women and confers some protection from conditions such as diabetes and ischaemic heart disease.

The complications of obesity affect all physiological systems (Figure 27.2). *Obese patients have increased morbidity and mortality from anaesthesia and surgery.*

Respiratory system
Obstructive sleep apnoea (OSA)

Patients with OSA experience periods of apnoea (greater than 10 seconds) and hypoventilation during sleep, with resultant desaturation and/or wakening. It is due to loss of pharyngeal tone when asleep and is exacerbated by alcohol and sedative drugs. OSA is more common in obese patients (60–90% of OSA sufferers are obese) and middle-aged men with BMI >30 and collar size >16.5". Symptoms are excessive snoring and daytime somnolence. Physiological changes occur – hypoxia, hypercapnia, polycythaemia and right ventricular hypertrophy.

OSA patients have an increased incidence of difficult intubation and a worsening of symptoms postoperatively due to CNS depressant drugs used during general anaesthesia.

Difficult intubation

Factors leading to difficult intubation include an increase in upper airway soft tissues, large tongue, fat face and cheeks, and a short fat neck. Neck mobility and mouth opening may also be reduced. Large breasts may hamper laryngoscope insertion.

Ventilation

Bag mask ventilation may be more difficult due to increased mass on the chest as well as increased abdominal pressure being displaced towards the head in an anesthetized and supine patient.

Obese patients have a reduced functional residual capacity (FRC). In health, the closing capacity (lung volume after small airway collapse) is less than FRC. In obese patients the closing capacity encroaches on FRC even when awake. Mass loading and diaphragmatic splinting also result in a reduction in total lung capacity and expiratory reserve volume. When anaesthetized, there is resultant right to left shunting, V/Q mismatch, arterial hypoxaemia and atelectasis (Figure 27.3).

Cardiovascular system

The main causes of morbidity and mortality from obesity are ischaemic heart disease, hypertension and cardiac failure.

Hypertension is more common with obesity: 50–60% of obese patients have mild to moderate hypertension, 5–10% have severe hypertension. For every 10 kg weight gain, the systolic/diastolic pressures increase by 3–4 mmHg and 2 mmHg, respectively. There is an increase in extracellular volume and cardiac output, left ventricular hypertrophy and reduced left ventricular function in response to exercise.

Cardiac dysrhythmias are more common due to hypoxia, hypercapnia, myocardial hypertrophy and conduction system infiltration.

Other factors

Gastrointestinal system Hiatus herniae are more common, with increased risk of regurgitation and aspiration of gastric contents, especially if abdominal pressure is increased by a large abdomen in the supine position. In extreme cases, lateral tilt may need to be employed to prevent aortocaval compression.

Endocrine Insulin resistance and Type 2 diabetes are more common.

Intravenous access This might prove difficult, potentially needing central venous access.

Positioning Particular attention must be paid to this. Extra supports may be needed and care taken with pressure points. Operating tables have a maximum weight (e.g. 150 kg). Hoists may have to be employed to transfer an anesthetized patient.

Anaesthetic management

Epidural or spinal anaesthesia should be considered if possible as they will avoid many, but not all, of the problems associated with general anaesthesia in an obese patient (e.g. aspiration risk, difficult intubation, hypoxia, etc.). In very large patients this might be difficult to achieve.

It might be preferable to induce anaesthesia in the operating theatre to obviate the problems of patient transfer. An appropriately sized BP cuff must be used (if the cuff is too small then the BP will read artificially high). If appropriate, a regional technique (e.g. nerve block, field block) should be considered, although, again, this may be more difficult to perform.

Very obese patients should have their airway secured with an endotracheal tube due to the risk of gastric content regurgitation, upper airway obstruction and the potential for hypoxia as a result of abnormal respiratory mechanics when they are anaesthetized. A reverse Trendelenburg position has been shown to aid intubation.

On emergence they must be extubated awake and in control of their own airway. They should be sitting up so as to reduce the work of breathing and increase their FRC.

Care must be taken with drugs causing sedation in the perioperative period due to their respiratory depressant effect and airway obstruction potential.

Drug doses are normally expressed in terms of dose per kg for normal-weight patients. The calculation of drug dosages in obese patients is complicated by the fact that, depending on the type of drug, the volume of distribution and rate of elimination will vary according to the degree of obesity – the dose of highly lipophilic drugs tends to be calculated on the basis of IBW, weakly lipophilic drugs are calculated on lean body mass, that is $(1 - \text{fat fraction}) \times$ kg.

Particular care with thomboprophylaxis is required for obese patients as they are at increased risk of both deep vein thrombosis and pulmonary embolism. They must therefore receive both drug (anticoagulant) and non-drug (e.g. compression stocking) prophylaxis.

Surgery for the treatment of obesity (bariatric) is becoming increasingly practised. Laparoscopic gastric banding as well as gastric bypass operations are performed. All the issues described in this chapter apply in these cases. Rapid weight loss can follow, as well as reversal of conditions such as diabetes and hypertension.

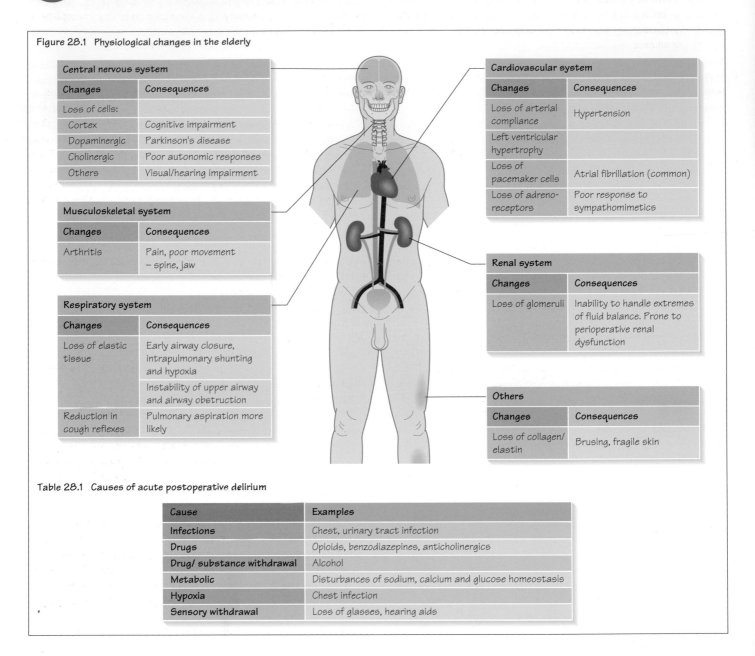

Figure 28.1 Physiological changes in the elderly

Central nervous system

Changes	Consequences
Loss of cells:	
Cortex	Cognitive impairment
Dopaminergic	Parkinson's disease
Cholinergic	Poor autonomic responses
Others	Visual/hearing impairment

Musculoskeletal system

Changes	Consequences
Arthritis	Pain, poor movement – spine, jaw

Respiratory system

Changes	Consequences
Loss of elastic tissue	Early airway closure, intrapulmonary shunting and hypoxia
	Instability of upper airway and airway obstruction
Reduction in cough reflexes	Pulmonary aspiration more likely

Cardiovascular system

Changes	Consequences
Loss of arterial compliance	Hypertension
Left ventricular hypertrophy	
Loss of pacemaker cells	Atrial fibrillation (common)
Loss of adreno-receptors	Poor response to sympathomimetics

Renal system

Changes	Consequences
Loss of glomeruli	Inability to handle extremes of fluid balance. Prone to perioperative renal dysfunction

Others

Changes	Consequences
Loss of collagen/ elastin	Brusing, fragile skin

Table 28.1 Causes of acute postoperative delirium

Cause	Examples
Infections	Chest, urinary tract infection
Drugs	Opioids, benzodiazepines, anticholinergics
Drug/ substance withdrawal	Alcohol
Metabolic	Disturbances of sodium, calcium and glucose homeostasis
Hypoxia	Chest infection
Sensory withdrawal	Loss of glasses, hearing aids

Projected demographic changes in the UK will result in an increase in the overall population, with the group over 75 years old growing fastest. Over the next 25 years this age group is projected to increase by 75%.

Anaesthesia for the elderly presents a challenge due to the decline in physiological reserves. For many physiological systems this reduction, and indeed loss of reserve, may not be apparent. Although there is recognition that biological age rather than chronological age is probably more relevant, there are nevertheless a number of changes that take place during the ageing process; in particular, cell loss (including loss of elastic tissue) and progression of common diseases (such as ischaemic heart disease and arthritis).

The impact of some of these changes is shown in Figure 28.1. Undertaking preoperative assessment is similar for all adults, but testing of physiological reserve is not always easy. For example, exercise tolerance may not be limited by cardiorespiratory reserve but by other factors such as arthritis. All patients should have serum electrolytes, glucose and a full blood count and an ECG. Further tests are as dictated by the patient's clinical findings and/or severity of surgery (e.g. major vascular surgery) but may include echocardiography, pharmacological stress testing, cardiopulmonary exercise testing, chest X ray and arterial blood gases. In addition, elderly patients will need a neurological assessment (e.g. the Mini-mental State Examination (MMSE)). This may help in the assessment of the patient's ability to give consent as well as understanding other processes (e.g. the use of PCA postoperatively).

Another key area is anaesthetic drug handling in the elderly. Changes in both pharmacokinetics and pharmacodynamics can lead to altered

Anaesthesia at a Glance, First Edition. Julian Stone and William Fawcett.

responses. Many drugs, such as opioids and i.v. anaesthetics, have a longer duration of action. This, together with a reduction in protein binding, results in a greater free (active) percentage of the drug, which can lead to inadvertent overdose. In addition, the markedly increased arm–brain circulation time may also trap the unwary anaesthetist into giving an excess dose of induction agent or sedative drugs. There is also a reduction in the MAC value of inhalational anaesthetics with increasing age, and so a lower concentration is required. For some drugs (e.g. β agonists) there is a reduced response, which may be important in the treatment of hypotension and during resuscitation.

Anaesthetic management of elderly patients

Preoperative care

The general principles of preoperative assessment are dealt with in Chapter 8. There are a few additional issues that are specifically related to caring for the elderly:

- Consent: has the patient understood the procedure and the alternatives? There may be concerns due to sensory deficit or poor cognition. Have family members and friends assisted if required? A separate form (called Consent Form 4) will be required for patients who lack capacity *and* if the procedure is in their best interests. This form may sometimes be signed by the family.
- Is surgery in the patient's best interests?
- For emergency admissions, there may be other hitherto unrecognized problems. For example if the patient has had a fall, is it due to confusion (e.g. chest or urinary infection), a cardiac dysrhythmia, aortic stenosis or a cerebrovascular event?

Induction of anaesthesia

Great care is required as the slow arm–brain circulation time, together with a poor response to vasopressors, may result in profound hypotension. Large-bore i.v. access will be required. Following loss of consciousness, maintaining the airway may be difficult as the soft tissues in the airway lose their tone. This problem is compounded in edentulous patients. Moreover, arthritic changes in the neck and jaw may make tracheal intubation difficult too.

General or regional?

Both techniques are used. With regional anaesthesia, the cardiovascular effects of hypotension (and with high blocks, bradycardia) may be resistant to drug treatment. Moreover, calcification in the ligaments of the back and difficulty in positioning of the patient may make the procedure technically difficult.

Fluid management

The general principles of fluid management are dealt with in Chapter 5. In the elderly, however, reduced physiological reserve can result in a very small therapeutic window for correct fluid management. Relatively small errors, either excess fluids (causing ventricular failure and oedema) or inadequate fluids (causing poor cardiac output, hypoten-sion and renal impairment) can have a large effect on outcome. Using simple markers to guide fluid therapy (pulse, blood pressure, urine output, capillary refill) may be inadequate and therefore central venous pressure and, more recently, flow measurements (e.g. oesophageal Doppler, see Chapter 3) are frequently used to guide fluid management, and in particular the response to fluid challenges.

Temperature

Maintenance of temperature is crucial. The elderly are more likely to become hypothermic (less fat) as well as less able to respond (reduced ability to vasoconstrict, shiver and increase metabolic rate). Hypothermia can be minimized by warming i.v. fluids and use of a warming mattress and forced air warmers over the patient peroperatively. Hypothermia causes a number of sequelae, such as reduced drug metabolism, increased vascular resistance, muscle weakness and coagulopathy. If shivering does occur it may increase oxygen consumption and lead to hypoxia.

Postoperative care (see Chapter 34)

Postoperatively, especially after major or emergency surgery, particular attention needs to be paid to:

- fluid management (as above);
- antibiotics (due to reduced immunity);
- anticoagulation (as there is risk of DVT and PE due to age, surgery and concurrent medical conditions);
- oxygen therapy (as above);
- pain control (this will require good assessment of pain; see below);
- nutrition (early enteral feeding if possible).

The following areas require specific mention:

- Acute postoperative delirium is not uncommon (Table 28.1).
- Postoperative cognitive dysfunction (POCD): elderly patients may suffer with this for days, weeks and even months postoperatively. The reasons may include cerebral emboli or metabolic disturbances. It may affect up to 25% of patients at 1 week and 10% at 3 months. Increasing age, infections, long operations and poor pre-existing cognitive function may all contribute.
- Response to postoperative events: the elderly mount a poor response or have reduced physical signs to infection, peritonitis (e.g. due to bowel anastomotic leak), haemorrhage, and myocardial ischaemia and pulmonary aspiration. All of these events may be silent in the early stages, and not become apparent until the patient is *in extremis*. There should be a low threshold to send patients to a high dependency or intensive care unit.
- Pain control: there are numerous problems with pain control including:
  - opioids – sedation and respiratory depression;
  - NSAIDs – GI bleeds and renal failure;
  - regional – hypotension.

Elderly patients require meticulous anaesthesia. Physiological reserve may be minimal and many problems may not be obvious until a late stage. Age itself is not a barrier to anaesthesia or intensive care treatment.

29 Anaesthesia and diabetes

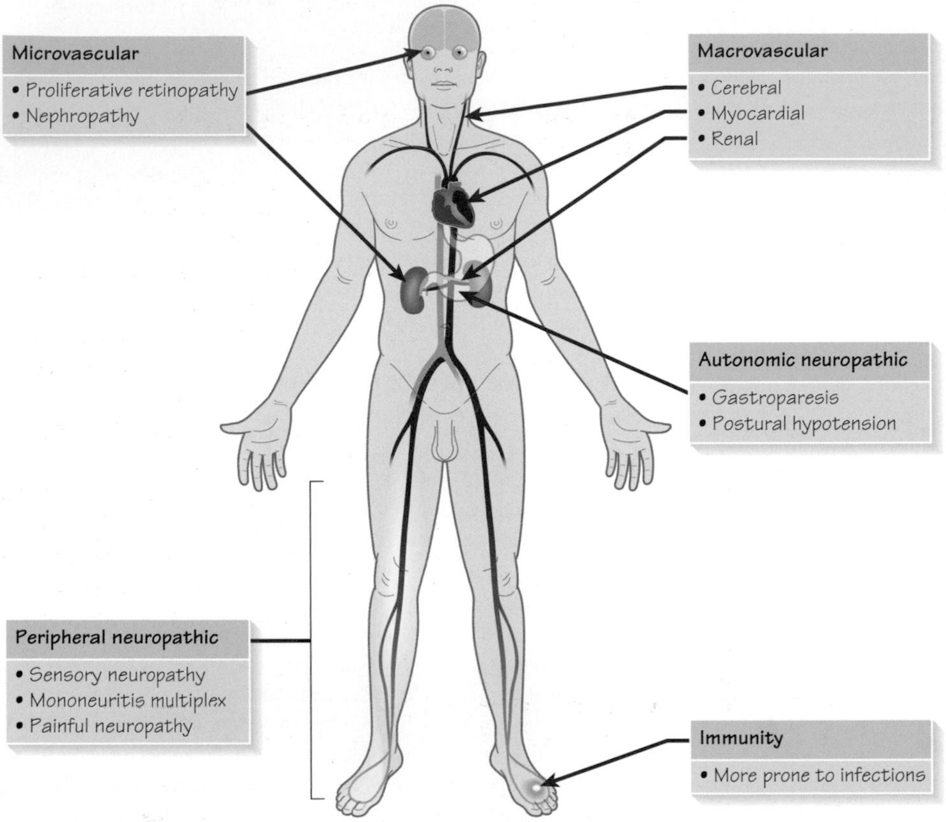

Figure 29.1 Complications of diabetes

Microvascular
- Proliferative retinopathy
- Nephropathy

Macrovascular
- Cerebral
- Myocardial
- Renal

Autonomic neuropathic
- Gastroparesis
- Postural hypotension

Peripheral neuropathic
- Sensory neuropathy
- Mononeuritis multiplex
- Painful neuropathy

Immunity
- More prone to infections

Table 29.2 Perioperative glycaemic control

Omit oral hypoglycaemics and normal s.c. insulin and use a GIK sliding scale with soluble insulin and 5% dextrose and KCl 20 mmol in 1 L, at 100 mL/h.

Initially test blood glucose 2 hourly and adjust as per the sliding scale:

Blood glucose (mmol/L)	Insulin (units/h)
0–4	0
5–9	1
10–14	2
15–19	3
>20	5

Table 29.1 Diabetes – key facts

	Type of diabetes	
	Type 1	**Type 2**
Aetiology	Beta cell destruction autoimmune, genetic, environmental (enterovirus)	Insulin hyposecretion ± insulin resistance
Clinical features	Tendency to ketosis	Ketosis rare. Obesity
Management	Insulin	May or may not require insulin
Diagnosis	Plasma glucose >11.1 mmol/L or a fasting >7.0 mmol/L	

Diabetes mellitus in patients undergoing major surgery poses a number of serious problems for the anaesthetist, particularly insulin-dependent diabetes. It is an independent predictor for serious postoperative complications such as perioperative myocardial infarction, renal failure, infections, mortality as well as length of hospital stay. In obstetrics, mothers with diabetes have a much higher incidence of stillbirth and congenital malformations. In addition, in the intensive care unit, for patients with and without diabetes, tight glycaemic control reduces both morbidity and mortality.

The key features of diabetes are shown in Table 29.1 and some of the major complications in Figure 29.1.

The essence of managing diabetes is to ensure good glycaemic control with rapid return to normal diet and medication. In addition, because of the potential for associated problems, especially vascular disease, patients need to be monitored for complications of this, such as myocardial ischaemia. Moreover, poor glycaemic control may precipitate diabetic ketoacidosis (DKA) or hyperosmolar non-ketotic coma (HONK), both of which carry a significant mortality. Many of the endocrine changes that occur following major surgery (e.g. increase in catecholamines, cortisol and glucagon) may increase blood glucose further (and indeed many patients without diabetes can have high blood glucose following major surgery).

Anaesthesia at a Glance, First Edition. Julian Stone and William Fawcett.

General management of blood glucose in patients with diabetes

Good glycaemic control may involve a good preoperative diet and weight loss, and perioperative insulin.

Insulin

This is required in the treatment for Type I diabetes. In addition, patients with Type 2 diabetes undergoing major surgery may need insulin.

There are three types of insulin:

* soluble insulin (rapid onset and short duration of action);
* intermediate duration of action;
* longer duration of action.

The latter two are insoluble as they are mixed with protamine or zinc to delay absorption, and can only be given subcutaneously. Patients are normally converted to soluble insulin preoperatively.

Type 2 diabetes can be managed with diet alone, with or without oral agents or insulin, depending on the degree of insulin resistance and background insulin secretion.

Management of blood glucose for diabetic patients undergoing surgery

Patients will require regular monitoring of their blood glucose perioperatively as follows:

* preoperatively;
* at least one peroperatively;
* in recovery.

In addition, patients on insulin initially require 2-hourly blood glucose measurement increasing to 4-hourly when stable. Non-insulin-dependent diabetes mellitus (NIDDM) patients require 8-hourly measurements.

Whilst hyperglycaemia is less dangerous than hypoglycaemia, 'permissive hyperglycaemia' is no longer acceptable, and blood glucose being kept between 6 and 10 mmol/L. Many patients with NIDDM will require insulin for major surgery as the stress response and concomitant insulin resistance will cause blood glucose levels to rise.

Insulin can be given intravenously according to two regimens. It is usually administered with glucose and potassium (so called GIK) unless the latter is high as dextrose and insulin alone will cause hypokalaemia. Insulin may be administered:

1 Separately according to a sliding scale with dextrose and potassium. The insulin rate is adjusted independently according to the blood glucose. This allows tight glucose control but runs the risk of hypoglycaemia if insulin is administered without dextrose (see Table 29.2).
2 Simultaneously with dextrose and potassium (Alberti regime). The amount of insulin in the bag is altered according to the blood glucose concentration. This ensures that insulin cannot be administered without glucose but may require frequent changes of bags with different insulin concentrations.

Patients should be first on the operating list to minimize fasting times and thus limit the chance of ketosis developing. It is convenient to classify surgery into minor (expecting to eat and drink in <4 hours) and major (all other surgery):

* For minor surgery omit oral hypoglycaemics and, for patients receiving insulin, give half dose of morning soluble insulin (if blood glucose >10 mmol/L) or no insulin (if blood glucose <10 mmol/L). Resume normal diet and medication as soon as possible afterwards. The blood glucose is checked peroperatively.
* For major surgery for all diabetics see Table 29.2.

General management of diabetic patients undergoing surgery

Other than the usual preoperative assessment (see Chapter 8) diabetic patients may also need assessment of potential problems:

* HbA1c (glycated haemoglobin) is a marker of glycaemic control over the last 2–3 months. A non-diabetic HbA1c is 3.5–5.5%. In patients with diabetes, 6.5% (48 mmol/mol) represents good control and >8% (64 mmol/mol) poor control, and thus more prone to microvascular complications. The measurements are changing soon to mmol/mol with 6.5% equivalent to 48 mmol/mol.
* Assessment of major diabetic complications, especially vascular. The degree of compromise from cardiovascular, cerebrovascular and renovascular impairment should be estimated from simple tests (e.g. serum urea and electrolytes) to more detailed investigations such as exercise testing, cardiac scans (echocardiography, thallium scanning, coronary angiography) and cerebrovascular scans (e.g. carotid duplex Doppler). Cardiac ischaemia may be silent due to autonomic neuropathy.

Conduct of anaesthesia

Attention should be focused on several key areas:

The airway Glycosylation of collagen in the cervical vertebrae and temporomandibular joints can cause difficulties in tracheal intubation.

Gastroparesis Patients with diabetes may have a delay in gastric emptying with autonomic neuropathy and may require tracheal intubation.

Regional anaesthesia Avoiding general anaesthesia with a quicker return to diet and medication is desirable but patients with diabetes may compensate poorly following sympathetic blockade and the infection risk (e.g. epidural abscess) is increased.

Infections These are more common and great care should be taken with any invasive procedures.

Postoperative care

The patient should return to their normal diet and medication as soon as possible. Careful postoperative care (e.g. HDU or ICU) with emphasis on oxygenation, fluid management with cardiovascular monitoring and infection control may lessen major complications.

Figure 30.1 (a) ECG: positive exercise test

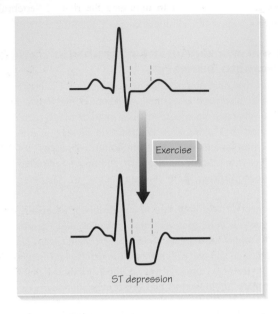

Exercise

ST depression

Figure 30.1 (b) Cardiopulmonary exercise testing (CPET)

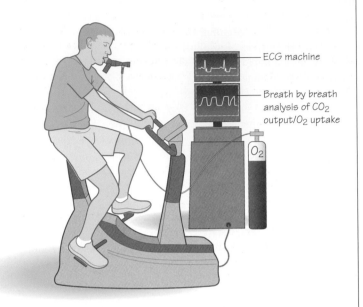

ECG machine

Breath by breath analysis of CO_2 output/O_2 uptake

Figure 30.1 (d) Pharmacological stress test

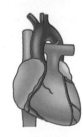

Heart scanning at rest or with pharmacological stress
- Dipyridamole–thallium scanning
- Dobutamine stress echocardiography

Figure 30.1 (c) Onset of anaerobic threshold determined by expired gas analysis

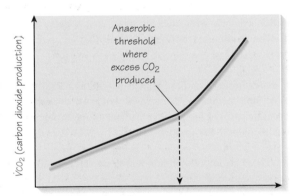

Anaerobic threshold where excess CO_2 produced

$\dot{V}CO_2$ (carbon dioxide production)

$\dot{V}O_2$ (oxygen consumption)

Positive dipyridamole–thallium scan, reversible perfusion defect

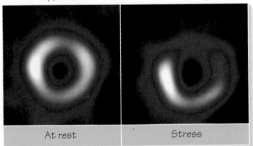

At rest | Stress

Table 30.1 Medication to reduce risk for patients undergoing vascular surgery

Drug	Comments
β blockers	• To help prevent ischaemia and arrhythmias • Avoid excessive dose (bradycardia and hypotension)
Statins	• Plaque stablization
ACE inhibitors	• For LV systolic dysfunction
Aspirin, warfarin and heparin	• After careful consideration of whether risk of haemorrhage outweighs risk of thrombosis

Anaesthesia at a Glance, First Edition. Julian Stone and William Fawcett.

74 © 2013 Julian Stone and William Fawcett. Published 2013 by John Wiley & Sons, Ltd.

Vascular surgery encompasses both ends of perioperative risks: arterial surgery, which is major, high-risk surgery, and venous surgery, which is very low-risk surgery, often performed under local anaesthesia. This chapter will focus on arterial surgery, which presents one of the biggest challenges for anaesthetists.

Arterial interventions place the patient at great risk of perioperative thrombosis and embolism. This is because the atherosclerotic process is generally widespread, affecting most major arteries. Moreover, given the high incidence in these patients of ischaemic heart disease, diabetes, renal dysfunction, cigarette smoking and increasing age, it becomes clear why this surgery presents such a high risk, with mortality or major cardiac complications of over 5%. The advent of less-invasive procedures may help in risk reduction (e.g. endovascular aneurysm repair [EVAR]).

Preoperative assessment

These patients require detailed assessment of physiological reserve. Many standard tests, such as ECG, are not very sensitive or specific and therefore exercise testing may be undertaken. However, these patients may not be able to exercise (e.g. due to claudication) thus testing reserve may be difficult.

Given that cardiac ischaemia and infarction accounts for the largest morbidity and mortality in this patient group, a full cardiac assessment is required. This may include:
- Resting and exercise ECG (Figure 30.1a).
- Cardiopulmonary exercise testing (CPET; Figure 30.1b) gives an objective assessment of reserve. Oxygen consumption and carbon dioxide production are measured. The point at which oxygen delivery becomes inadequate to meet energy demands of aerobic metabolism is called the anaerobic threshold (AT; Figure 30.1c). The oxygen consumption at the onset of supplementary anaerobic metabolism is described in mL/kg/min. An AT of less than 11 mL/kg/min implies greatly increased risk; if this is coupled with myocardial ischaemia the risk is even higher.
- If exercising is not possible, pharmacological stress tests may be used to assess coronary perfusion, such as dipyridamole–thallium scanning (Figure 30.1d) or dobutamine stress echocardiography.
- Echocardiography gives an assessment of left ventricular and valvular function (Figure 30.1d).
- Coronary angiography may be required prior to the vascular surgery to decide whether or not revascularization is required.

In addition, renovascular and cerebrovascular disease need to be quantified and the latter may also require surgery for severe (>70%) carotid stenosis.

Appropriate medication may also need to be instituted or continued (Table 30.1), together with life-style advice (e.g. cessation of smoking). Other co-morbidities will need to be optimized such as diabetes and chronic obstructive pulmonary disease.

Preoperative treatment

Monitoring The aim is to keep vascular parameters as near as possible to baseline values, with meticulous attention to oxygenation, heart rate and blood pressure control. In addition to standard monitoring, arterial and central venous pressure monitoring are used, and many would measure cardiac output too (e.g. oesophageal Doppler).

Temperature management Normothermia is important to prevent vasoconstriction, which will increase cardiac afterload. In addition, hypothermia reduces drug metabolism, will cause haemodynamic instability during rewarming and may cause arrhythmias, coagulopathy and shivering.

Analgesia A thoracic epidural provides excellent analgesia and increased flow from vasodilation. However, it is important to ensure that coagulation is normal to minimize the risk of vertebral canal haematoma.

Haemodynamic instability Prompt management of haemodynamic upset is required. This can occur during blood loss or during arterial clamping or unclamping. Vasoactive drugs to reduce blood pressure (e.g. nitrates) and increase blood pressure (e.g. phenylephrine) must be to hand.

Kidneys Renal impairment is a potential problem postoperatively and may require renal support. It is crucial that further insults are avoided (e.g. hypovolaemia, NSAIDs etc.).

Others Good glucose control and infection control are essential.

Postoperative care

Following major arterial surgery, patients should be transferred to a high dependency or intensive care unit for monitoring, with much of the above applicable to the postoperative period too.

Ruptured abdominal aortic aneurysm (AAA): a common vascular emergency

Ruptured AAA carries an overall mortality rate of 60% or more (compared to about 5% for elective repair). The blood bank should be alerted and the massive transfusion protocol instituted. Good peripheral venous access (two 14 G cannulae) attached to warmed i.v. fluids, as well as central venous and arterial access, are required. The major challenges are:
- massive blood loss and associated coagulopathy;
- end organ damage, particularly myocardial and renal;
- hypothermia and acidosis.

Induction of anaesthesia can cause catastrophic hypotension from vasodilation, loss of sympathetic tone and loss of abdominal wall tone. The patient should thus be draped and the surgeon ready to operate before induction commences. Blood products and vasoactive medication (including epinephrine) should be close at hand.

Once the aorta is clamped (which may cause a degree of hypertension and myocardial ischaemia) the patient is judiciously prepared in terms of blood volume, haemoglobin and coagulation for when the unclamping of the graft occurs. Great attention should be taken to warm all i.v. fluids and ensure normothermia (although the legs should not be warmed during the ischaemic phase to reduce their metabolic rate and limit ischaemic damage.) If there is profound acidosis (which carries a poor prognosis) many would treat with sodium bicarbonate if the pH <7.0.

Unclamping causes marked hypotension from hypovolaemia, and myocardial depression and vasodilation from acidosis. Hyperkalaemia can also occur. It is often wise for the surgeon to release the clamp intermittently.

Table 31.1 Predictors of difficult intubation (see Chapter 16)

History	• Surgery/radiotherapy to head and neck • Obstructive sleep apnoea (OSA) • Pregnancy • Conditions affecting tongue size • Conditions affecting neck mobility • Conditions affecting mouth opening
Examination	• Receding jaw • Protruding upper incisors • Large tongue • Large neck circumference • Obesity • Tumour/infection/trauma/swelling/burns and scarring of the airway
Tests	• Mouth opening • Mallamapati • Forward movement of jaw • Thyromental distance <6cm • Sternomental distance <12.5cm

Table 31.2 Airway devices used for surgery (see Chapter 4)

Device	Comments
Laryngeal mask airway (LMA), plain or reinforced	Ear, nose and facial surgery. Some use for tonsillectomy and dental extractions too. Can become dislodged. Provides good but not definitive protection from blood etc
Oral tracheal tube, usually preformed Ring–Adair–Elwyn tube (RAE tube)	Throat surgery. Definitive protection
Nasotracheal tube	Intraoral surgery
Microlaryngeal tube	Small tube to provide good access to vocal cords
Laser tube	Metallic tubes that are safe when lasers are used
Tracheostomy	For operations where the upper airway is obstructed or removed (laryngectomy)
None	Patient jet ventilated where the presence of a tube makes surgery impossible

Figure 31.1 Management of unexpected difficult airway

Laryngoscopy and tracheal intubation	Laryngeal mask airway insertion	Maintain oxygenation. Consider waking patient	Consider other approaches to airway e.g. fibre-optic intubation if safe to do so	Surgical access to airway: • Cricothyrotomy • Tracheostomy
if not	*if not*	*if not*	*if not*	

Figure 31.3 View of larynx from fibre-optic laryngoscope

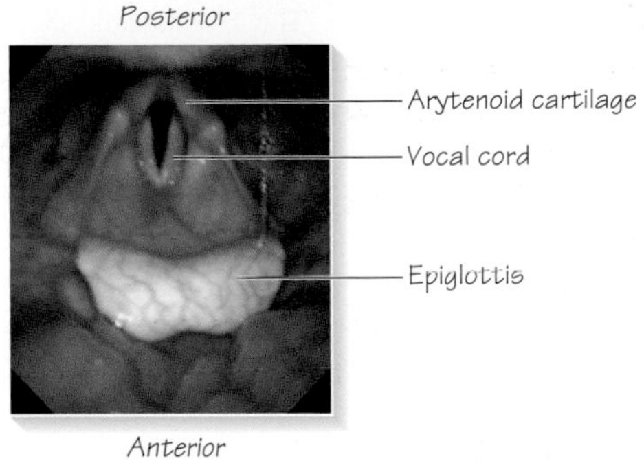

Posterior

— Arytenoid cartilage

— Vocal cord

— Epiglottis

Anterior

Figure 31.2

Anaesthetist undertaking fibre-optic laryngoscopy

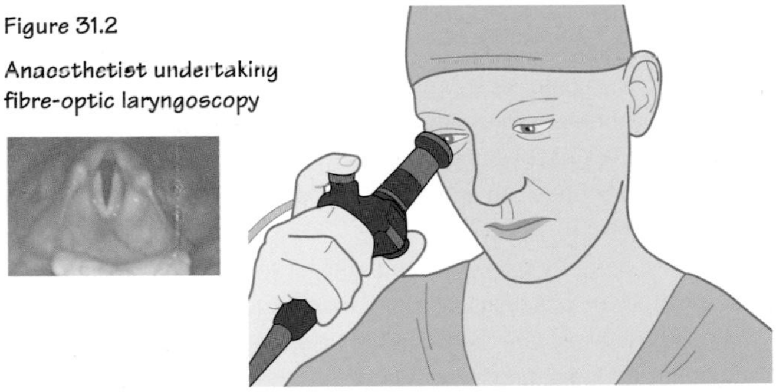

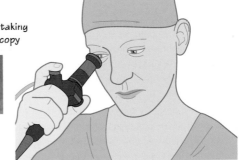

Table 31.3 Approaches to patient with known or difficult airway

Technique	Comments
Gaseous induction	Said to provide a safer induction as the patient will not breathe more anaesthetic should airway obstruction occur and necessitate waking up. Latter **cannot** be relied on.
Awake fibre-optic intubation	Allows the airway to be secured but difficult if blood or gross anatomical distortion present
Asleep fibre-optic intubation	More pleasant for patient but risk being unable to ventilate patient when unconscious
Tracheostomy	Can be performed under local anaesthetic for severe airway compromise

Table 31.4 Principles of care for patients undergoing freeflap surgery

Principle	Technique used
Maintain high cardiac output	Fluids, monitored by Doppler/LiDCO
Reduce systemic vascular resistance	Vasodilators
Normothermia	Active warming of patient and fluids
Reduce blood viscosity	Preventing hypothermia. Aim for haemoglobin of 100g/L (haemodilution)
Monitor flap blood flow	Doppler
Good analgesia	Local anaesthetics, opioids
Other precautions for prolonged surgery	Very careful positioning, eye care, DVT prophylaxis

Anaesthesia at a Glance, First Edition. Julian Stone and William Fawcett.

ENT and maxillofacial surgery present unique challenges to the anaesthetist. The proximity of the surgeon to the airway – sometimes in the airway itself – means that the anaesthetist and surgeon share the airway. Thus great cooperation is needed between the two. Access is often restricted due to surgical instruments or drapes. Moreover, the airway itself may be compromised during the operation from preexisting pathology (tumours/infection) or from blood, bone, etc.; therefore, meticulous assessment and management of the airway is required at all times. Protection of other structures, particularly the eyes, is also important as they may be wrapped in drapes too.

Many different operations are performed but only a few will be discussed here:
- ear: grommets, middle ear surgery;
- nasal: sinus surgery;
- throat: tonsillectomy, laryngsocopy, laryngectomy;
- maxillofacial: orthognathic surgery, free flap;
- emergency surgery: post-tonsillectomy haemorrhage, airway obstruction, trauma.

Preoperative assessment
The patient population comes from diverse groups: mainly children for some ENT procedures (e.g. tonsillectomy and grommets) and elderly patients, often with co-morbidities secondary to tobacco and alcohol, for throat tumours and free flap procedures.

Airway
The airway is clearly fundamental to all anaesthetic practice but is pivotal in the management of these patients. The topic is dealt with in Chapter 16, and is summarized in Table 31.1. Of particular importance to ENT patients are:
- A history of obstructive sleep apnoea (OSA), with some patients requiring continuous positive airway pressure (CPAP) at night. These patients may require care in an HDU postoperatively, with monitoring of oxygen saturation.
- A history of difficult intubation in the past, although surgery, radiotherapy or tumour progression may change the situation.
- Stridor: this implies at least 50% reduction in the airway diameter and requires senior skilled input until the airway is secured or the obstruction removed or bypassed.

Peroperative considerations
Safe management of the airway is crucial. The use of airway devices and approaches to difficult airways are shown in Tables 31.2 and 31.3 and Figures 31.1, 31.2 and 31.3.
- **Ear surgery**:
  - Insertion of grommets is often performed in young children. The head is turned and tube dislodgement may occur.
  - Middle ear surgery: often induced hypotension is used to facilitate surgery. The surgeon may use facial nerve monitoring and as a result neuromuscular blocking drugs may have to be avoided.

- **Nasal surgery**:
  - An LMA is often used for sinus surgery. Topical preparation of the nasal mucosa is often used (e.g. Moffat's solution, containing adrenaline and cocaine). Great care is required here as inadvertent i.v. injection can be fatal. Again, induced hypotension may be used.
- **Throat surgery**:
  - Tonsillectomy can be performed with either a tracheal tube or LMA. In small children beware blood loss, which can be a significant proportion of their total blood volume.
  - Laryngeal surgery will require specialized airway control (Table 31.2), depending on the surgery, and patients may have difficult airways. Patients undergoing laryngectomy will require a peroperative tracheostomy.
- **Maxillofacial surgery**:
  - dental extraction (see Chapter 33);
  - orthognathic surgery – this is for altering position of jaw bones, e.g. mandibular osteotomy;
  - free flap surgery (see below).

Special areas
Reducing blood loss
Some operations require blood loss to be reduced preoperatively to improve the operating field, often by reducing arterial and venous pressure. Great care is required to ensure that end organ damage (myocardial and cerebral) does not result. Drugs used include β blockers, vasodilators and centrally acting drugs (e.g. clonidine). The blood pressure will need to be restored prior to the end of surgery to ensure that haemostasis is adequate.

Laser surgery
Laser surgery presents a major potential hazard – an airway fire. Standard tracheal tubes will melt and with oxygen provides the perfect conditions for combustion, which carries a high mortality. These patients require a laser-safe tube, often a flexometallic tube.

Free flap surgery (Table 31.4)
Free flap surgery involves the transfer of a block of tissue with its own blood supply from a remote site to the primary site of surgery.

Emergency surgery
Post-tonsillectomy haemorrhage
This is a serious problem in a child who may be hypovolaemic and have a stomach full of blood. Meticulous airway management and fluid resuscitation (sometimes with blood) may be required.

Airway obstruction (Table 31.4)
Patients may present with stridor. Heliox (a mixture of, usually, 79% helium and 21% oxygen) can be used as it is less dense than air and causes less turbulence in the airway. A variety of techniques can be used to secure the airway (Table 31.3), including a tracheostomy under LA.

32 Awareness

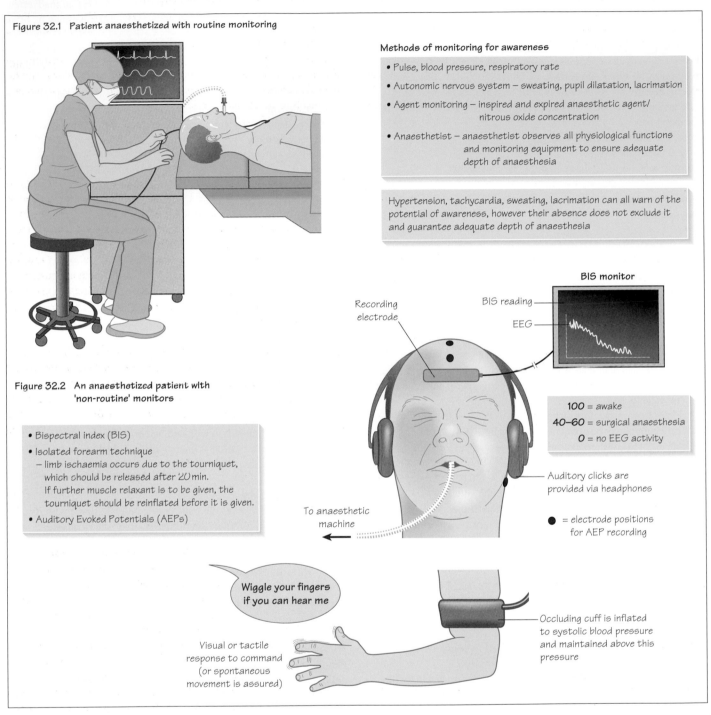

Figure 32.1 Patient anaesthetized with routine monitoring

Methods of monitoring for awareness

- Pulse, blood pressure, respiratory rate
- Autonomic nervous system – sweating, pupil dilatation, lacrimation
- Agent monitoring – inspired and expired anaesthetic agent/ nitrous oxide concentration
- Anaesthetist – anaesthetist observes all physiological functions and monitoring equipment to ensure adequate depth of anaesthesia

Hypertension, tachycardia, sweating, lacrimation can all warn of the potential of awareness, however their absence does not exclude it and guarantee adequate depth of anaesthesia

BIS monitor

BIS reading

EEG

Recording electrode

Figure 32.2 An anaesthetized patient with 'non-routine' monitors

- Bispectral index (BIS)
- Isolated forearm technique
  – limb ischaemia occurs due to the tourniquet, which should be released after 20 min. If further muscle relaxant is to be given, the tourniquet should be reinflated before it is given.
- Auditory Evoked Potentials (AEPs)

100 = awake
40–60 = surgical anaesthesia
0 = no EEG activity

Auditory clicks are provided via headphones

● = electrode positions for AEP recording

To anaesthetic machine

Wiggle your fingers if you can hear me

Visual or tactile response to command (or spontaneous movement is assured)

Occluding cuff is inflated to systolic blood pressure and maintained above this pressure

Awareness is an issue of major concern for both the anaesthetist and patient and is often brought up preoperatively as an area of anxiety by patients.

The most extreme form of awareness is the paralysed patient who experiences pain and is unable to alert anyone to their situation. This has been likened to torture, with a significant incidence of post-traumatic stress disorder. Thankfully this is very rare, in part due to:
- the reduced use of muscle relaxants – spontaneously breathing patients can still experience awareness but since they are not paralysed they are able to move, which will alert the anaesthetist to the problem;
- improvements in patient and anaesthetic monitoring;
- increased appreciation of awareness.

There are different types of awareness:
- **Conscious awareness with spontaneous or prompted recall** (explicit recall): in this type, specific events or conversations are recalled by the patient after the operation.

Anaesthesia at a Glance, First Edition. Julian Stone and William Fawcett.

- **Conscious awareness with amnesia**: patients are able to respond to command during anaesthesia (e.g. to move a finger) but have no recollection afterwards.
- **Dreaming**: this might occur during anaesthesia and in the postoperative period.
- **Unconscious awareness** (implicit recall): events or suggestions might be recollected under hypnosis postoperatively as well as behaviour modification (e.g. instructions given to the patient during their anaesthetic, such as to touch their ear, might be replicated after hospital discharge when exposed to the appropriate stimulus).

The incidence of awareness has been reported to range between 0.2% and 1.6% in surgical patients. Of this group:
- 8% were in Caesarean sections;
- 45% were in emergency surgery (inadequate anaesthetic depth);
- 10% of patients who reported awareness experienced pain.

During life-saving emergency surgery, inadequate anaesthesia could potentially occur if the cardiovascular depressant effects of the anaesthetic impacted on the adequacy of coronary and cerebral perfusion pressure.

Anaesthesia is likely to affect the memory of awareness rather than the actual awareness itself.

Causes of awareness

Analysis of Medical Defence Union (UK) claims of awareness for a single year showed 70% of episodes were due to faulty technique and 20% were due to failure to check equipment. Only 2.5% of claims were due to equipment failure, unknown causes, spurious claims or justified risks (e.g. in critically ill patients).

End-tidal anaesthetic agent monitoring is one of the minimum standards required when any patient is anaesthetized (Figure 32.1). The expired concentration of volatile anaesthetic relates to the amount given as well as brain concentration, although it does not in itself measure the extent of anaesthesia. Monitoring the minimum alveolar concentration of an exhaled volatile anaesthetic agent confirms that the patient received the drug but it does not confirm or guarantee lack awareness. Also, no account is taken of the physiological response of the patient or the effect of surgical stimulation.

There is interdependence between hypnosis, analgesia and the degree of surgical stimulation to which a patient is exposed. Premedication, interoperative analgesia and anaesthetic nerve blocks all reduce the degree of hypnotic needed to prevent awareness and so these variables, as well as the physiological response to surgery, must be taken into account for each individual when anaesthetizing patients.

Patients at risk of awareness

Although any patient undergoing anaesthesia has the potential to experience awareness, those at high risk include:
- a previous history of awareness;
- difficult intubation including protracted attempts to perform this procedure;
- emergency surgery in shocked/critically ill patients;
- obstetric patients;
- cardiac surgery.

Methods of assessment and measurement

There is no single technique, set of clinical data or piece of equipment that is perfect for the monitoring and detection of awareness, although currently bispectral index monitoring is popular (Figure 32.2). Autonomic changes that are monitored include:

- Pupil size and reactivity, although these are unreliable indicators. Pupil mydriasis may be caused by anticholinergics (e.g. atropine, hyoscine), whilst opiates cause miosis.
- Changes in blood pressure, although these may be related to other factors, such as circulating catecholamines and drugs (e.g. beta blockers) and there is no consistent relationship between blood pressure and the patient's level of consciousness.
- Heart rate variability: reports suggest that there is a reduction in respiratory sinus arrhythmia with anaesthesia. In normal sinus arrhythmia the heart rate increases on inspiration and decreases on expiration as a result of variations in preload.
- Sweating and lacrimation are also warnings of awareness.

Current methods available to monitor awareness include the following:

Isolated forearm technique An arm blood pressure cuff is inflated and maintained above systolic BP at the onset of anaesthesia. This is done before any systemic neuromuscular blocking drug is given, thereby leaving the limb distal to the cuff unaffected and able to mount a motor response if attempted. Movement, either spontaneous or in response to command, can then be observed. A patient might respond to command, for example to move a finger, without having postoperative recall. It is mainly used as a research tool. Limb ischaemia caused by the tourniquet occurs and the adequacy of motor response is insufficient after 20 minutes.

Electroencephalogram (EEG) Whilst not practical to be used routinely (both in terms of equipment and interpretation) the overall pattern of EEG reading whilst anaesthetized shows similarities with different anaesthetic agents. With increasing depth of anaesthesia there is an increase in average wave amplitude and a decrease in average frequency. There is also a progressive change from beta to delta waveform.

Bispectral index (BIS) This is a simplified EEG which uses an algorithm that converts EEG signals into an index of hypnotic level, ranging from 0 = no EEG activity to 100 = awake. A figure of 40–60 is recommended for general anaesthesia.

Evoked potentials Whilst the EEG incorporates the response of thousands of neurons across the cerebral cortex, evoked potentials record the response of a far smaller and more localized group of neurons (e.g. brainstem, midbrain, cerebral cortex) to a specific stimulus or set of stimuli. The signals are time-locked and then averaged in order to limit other EEG components such as random noise.
- Auditory-evoked potentials: electrical activity passing from the cochlea to auditory cortex in response to stimulus is recorded. EEG analysis shows characteristic waveforms whose amplitude decreases and latency increases with depth of anaesthesia. This correlates well with transition from sleep to awake but is a poor predictor of response to painful stimuli.
- Visual-evoked potentials: the patient wears goggles with light-emitting diodes lying within them. The flashing diodes create visual-evoked potentials, which are detected and recorded over the visual cortex. This may be useful for assessing sedation in intensive care patients.
- Somatosensory-evoked potentials: stimuli are placed peripherally (e.g. median nerve) and the response is recorded over the cervical vertebrae and the contralateral somatosensory cortex. Each calculation takes over 1 minute and results are inconsistent.

33 Anaesthesia for ECT, dental surgery and special needs

Figure 33.1 ECT bite block

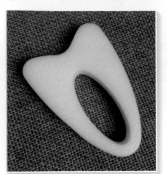

Table 33.1 Physiological and clinical effects of ECT

Physiological effect	Clinical effect
Cardiovascular:	
• Parasympathetic tone increased (early)	Bradycardia, asystole
• Sympathetic tone increased (late)	Tachycardia, hypertension
Cerebral:	
• Increase in oxygen consumption, blood flow and ICP	May provoke TIA, haemorrhage, status epilepticus
• ? Cerebral damage	Cognitive impairment

Figure 33.2 Hazards in chair dental surgery

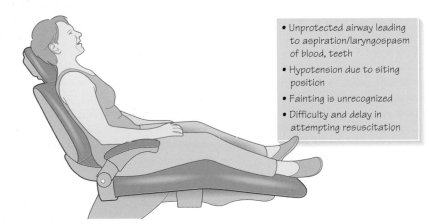

- Unprotected airway leading to aspiration/laryngospasm of blood, teeth
- Hypotension due to siting position
- Fainting is unrecognized
- Difficulty and delay in attempting resuscitation

Anaesthesia for electroconvulsive therapy

Electroconvulsive therapy (ECT) is used mainly for severe depression, where other treatments have failed. It involves passing a current through the brain, inducing a fit. Generally, four to six treatments are administered twice weekly during a course of therapy. There are various immediate side effects, including headache and short-term memory loss, but there may be long-term cognitive effects as well. Usually, bilateral ECT is used as it seems more effective but unilateral ECT may have fewer side effects. There is debate about the optimum fit duration, with too short (<10 seconds) and too long (2 minutes) being less effective.

There are a number of considerations for the anaesthetist undertaking anaesthesia for ECT.

Remote location

ECT very often takes place in remote psychiatric units and the presence of a senior anaesthetist is mandatory. As with any anaesthetic, full precautions are mandatory and include oxygen, suction, monitoring and full resuscitation equipment and drugs.

Consent

Most patients can give consent but sometimes ECT may take place under the Mental Health Act.

Co-morbidities

Patients are often elderly with other co-morbidities. A full history (which may prove to be impossible) and examination should take place. Sometimes ECT should be postponed to improve the patients physical status (e.g. heart failure) but this has to be weighed up against the risk of delaying treatment. ECT should not be administered if the patient has had a recent myocardial infarction, cerebrovascular accident or has raised intracranial pressure or a cerebral aneurysm. If the patient has a pacemaker or an automated implantable cardioverter-defibrillator (AICD) then cardiological assistance should be sought. Occasionally, patients may need to be transferred to an acute hospital with the psychiatrist and ECT machine to allow safe administration of ECT.

The anaesthetic

The patient receives an induction agent and, to minimize adverse effects from the convulsion such as tongue biting and even fractures and dislocations (e.g. jaw and, historically, spine), a short-acting muscle relaxant is given. The patient then has a bite block inserted (Figure 33.1), to protect the teeth, lips and tongue, and the ECT is delivered. The anaesthetist ventilates the patient with a facemask until respirations resume and the patient is transferred to the recovery area.

There has been much debate about the use of different induction agents and muscle relaxants. Until the advent of propofol, methohexi-

Anaesthesia at a Glance, First Edition. Julian Stone and William Fawcett.

tone (a barbiturate) was commonly used but today the most common anaesthetic is propofol and suxamethonium (the latter in a reduced dose).

Physiological effects of ECT
These are shown in Table 33.1.

Anaesthesia for dental surgery
Most dental surgery is performed under local anaesthesia, but difficult extractions, or surgery in young patients, severely phobic patients or those patients with special needs (see below) will require general anaesthesia. This is very stimulating surgery and can cause both bradycardia and asystole as well as tachyarrhythmias (mediated via the V cranial nerve). Many of the principles are covered in Chapter 31. The key areas are as follows.

Shared airway
Close cooperation with the surgeon is required as the surgeon is operating around the airway. Historically, patients underwent nasotracheal intubation with a throat pack, which provided definitive airway control and protection. However, more recently, many units undertake this surgery with an LMA alone, which provides good conditions but great care needs to be exercised to ensure the LMA does not become dislodged.

Protection of the airway
Any dental surgery has the potential for blood and bone fragments to enter the pharynx and hence the airway. If an LMA is used the surgeon will generally protect against this with swabs and suction.

Difficult airways
Some patients with acute dental infections requiring extractions may have severe trismus. In these cases consideration will have to be given to fibre-optic nasotracheal intubation, either awake or under sedation, or under general anaesthesia, depending on the circumstances.

Chair dental surgery
Once commonly performed in dental surgeries, with hypoxic anaesthetic mixtures and little or no monitoring, these procedures are now much less commonly performed. If this is carried out, they are undertaken in an environment where full monitoring and resuscitation are available. The type of surgery performed in the dental chair under anaesthesia is usually quick dental extractions, typically deciduous teeth in children. The patient is sat up and a mask is applied over the nose whilst the surgeon operates. There are a number of issues, as shown in Figure 33.2.

Anaesthesia for those with special needs
Special needs encompasses a large spectrum of diagnoses, including learning, psychological, psychiatric and medical disorders. There may be a number of issues for these patients.

Consent
Patients may be able to understand and give consent for any proposed procedure or they may require someone to give consent on their behalf.

Co-morbidities
In some circumstances the special need may be an isolated phenomenon, in others it may be part of a syndrome (e.g. Down's) associated with epilepsy, cardiac disease, cervical spine instability, etc. Obtaining a history may not be possible and the patient's carers and/or GP are invaluable in this respect.

Conduct of anaesthesia
The type of anaesthetic and other areas such as regional blockade or use of PCA will depend on the patients ability to understand and cooperate. Some patients with severe physical disabilities may have very poorly developed peripheral veins and hence venous access may be very difficult.

Proposed surgery
Some patients may have surgery that is unfamiliar to the anaesthetist (e.g. restorative dentistry) and close cooperation with the surgeon will be required.

Figure 34.1 Side effects of opioids

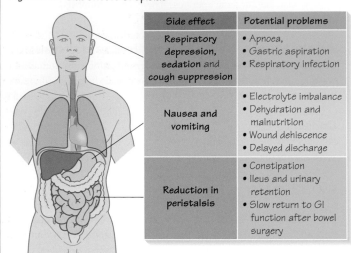

Side effect	Potential problems
Respiratory depression, sedation and cough suppression	• Apnoea, • Gastric aspiration • Respiratory infection
Nausea and vomiting	• Electrolyte imbalance • Dehydration and malnutrition • Wound dehiscence • Delayed discharge
Reduction in peristalsis	• Constipation • Ileus and urinary retention • Slow return to GI function after bowel surgery

Table 34.1 Drugs used for multimodal analgesia

Drug	Side effects
Opioids	See Figure 34.1
NSAIDs	• Bleeding, especially gastrointestinal • Gastrointestinal perforation • Asthma, renal failure • Myocardial and cerebral thrombosis
Paracetamol	• Liver dysfunction in overdose
Local anaesthetics	• Cardiac and CNS toxicity

Table 34.2 Common methods of administering analgesics

Analgesic	Method
Opioids	i.m., i.v. (PCA), epidural/spinal, oral, intra-articular
Paracetamol	i.v. and oral (rarely p.r.)
NSAIDs	Oral, p.r., i.v.
Local anaesthetic	Wound, epidural/spinal, various nerve blocks. Intra-articular

Table 34.3 Levels of postoperative care

Level of care	
0 (ward)	Patients needs met on normal ward
1 (HDU)	Patients at risk of their condition deteriorating, or who require advice from the ICU team
2 (ICU)	Patients with a single failing organ system or requiring detailed observation/intervention
3 (ICU)	Patients requiring ventilation (alone), advanced respiratory support alone or support of at least two organ systems

Table 34.4 Modified early warning score

Score	3	2	1	0	1	2	3
CNS	Confused agitated			Alert	Responds to voice	Responds to pain	Unresponsive
Respiratory (breaths per min)	<8			8–20	21–30		>30
Heart rate (beats per min)	<40		41–50	51–100	101–110	111–130	>130
Systolic BP (mmHg)	<70	71–80	81–100	101–180	181–200	201–220	>220
Temperature (°C)	<34	34–35		35.1–37.5	37.6–38.5	38.6–40	>40
S_aO_2 (%)	<90	91–93		94–100			
Urine output (2h) (mL/h)	<30						

Figure 34.2 Hazards of postoperative hypoxaemia

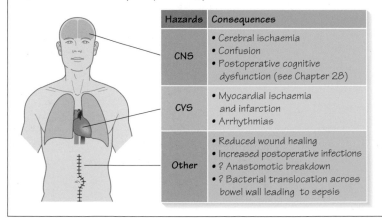

Hazards	Consequences
CNS	• Cerebral ischaemia • Confusion • Postoperative cognitive dysfunction (see Chapter 28)
CVS	• Myocardial ischaemia and infarction • Arrhythmias
Other	• Reduced wound healing • Increased postoperative infections • ? Anastomotic breakdown • ? Bacterial translocation across bowel wall leading to sepsis

Figure 34.3 Venturi effect

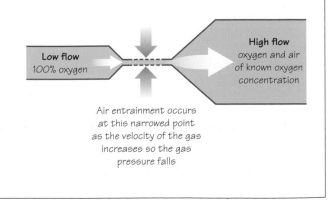

Low flow 100% oxygen

High flow oxygen and air of known oxygen concentration

Air entrainment occurs at this narrowed point as the velocity of the gas increases so the gas pressure falls

Anaesthesia at a Glance, First Edition. Julian Stone and William Fawcett.

The role of the anaesthetist is not limited to theatres. There may be a number of postoperative responsibilities to undertake, both in the recovery room and on the surgical ward.

Analgesia

Multimodal analgesia is used, which works on the principle that drugs acting by different mechanisms can result in additive or synergistic analgesia with lowered adverse effects. In particular there is an attempt to minimize opioids ('opioid sparing') to reduce their adverse effects (Figure 34.1).

Some of the different drugs that have been used are shown in Table 34.1. The mainstay of analgesia is paracetamol, non-steroidal anti-inflammatory drugs (NSAIDs), local anaesthetics and opioids. Safety is paramount in pain management. Most pain is self-limiting, with analgesic requirements falling by 48 hours, even after major surgery.

A practical approach uses the WHO three step analgesic ladder (see Chapter 13). Simple analgesics should be tried (e.g. NSAIDs and paracetamol), then mild opioids (e.g. codeine, tramadol) and finally strong opioids (e.g. morphine). Regular administration affords better pain control than p.r.n. (as required) administration.

Common methods of administering drugs are listed in Table 34.2. For major surgery the use of infusion devices such as PCAs, epidurals or local anaesthetic infusions around major nerves (e.g. paravertebral/brachial plexus) are used.

Fluids

Patients will require i.v. fluids until they are able to drink normally (see Chapter 5). For some patients no i.v. fluids are required, for others i.v. fluids will be required for several days.

Fluid is required for the following:
- maintenance and interoperative fluid losses;
- replacement of pre-existing losses (e.g. dehydration preoperatively);
- replacement of postoperative losses (e.g. nasogastric losses, bleeding).

The types of fluid are:
- isotonic crystalloid (most often used);
- colloids (for maintaining intravascular volume, early bleeding);
- blood and blood products (for significant haemorrhage, coagulopathy).

Other than maintenance fluids (approximately 2.5 L/day with 50–100 mmol/day of sodium and 40–80 mmol/day of potassium), fluids are prescribed to replace the composition of the fluid lost.

A fluid challenge is sometimes administered to patients with a low urine output, hypotension, low CVP or stroke volume. Typically, 250 mL of colloid is given and any response (i.e. a significant increase in the above measurements) suggests the patient had a reduced intravascular volume. The fluid challenge is repeated until no further increase occurs. Flow-directed measurements may also be used (Chapter 5).

Negligible calories are present in i.v. fluids and therefore if patients are unable to eat or tolerate enteral feed (e.g. from a jejunal tube) for a prolonged period, parenteral nutrition (i.v. feeding) will be required.

Referral to high dependency unit/intensive care unit

Postoperatively, some patients require more clinical input on a high dependency unit (HDU) or an intensive care unit (ICU). Common definitions and examples of levels of care are given in Table 34.3. Usually, the precise level of care is determined preoperatively but occasionally unplanned admissions to ICU are required. This may be a result of major blood loss, sepsis or an exacerbation of pre-existing medical conditions such as an MI.

Early warning scores (EWS)

EWS assist in early detection of the deteriorating patient, allowing early management and improved outcome. It is a simple physiological scoring system (Table 34.4). When the score reaches 3 (some use 4 or even 5, but certainly 3 in a single category), this triggers a review of the patient at senior level. In addition, a repeat score assesses any intervention (e.g. oxygenation and i.v. fluids). Various EWS exist, including a modified EWS (MEWS) and an obstetric MEWS (MEOWS).

Oxygen therapy

Following sedation, all patients breathing room air will have varying degrees of hypoxaemia, as the increase in arterial CO_2 pressure (P_aCO_2) will necessarily cause a decrease in alveolar O_2 pressure (P_{AO_2}) and therefore arterial PO_2. This is embodied in the alveolar gas equation:

$$P_{AO_2} \propto F_iO_2 - (P_aCO_2 / RQ)$$

where RQ is the respiratory quotient.

Although increasing P_aCO_2 reduces P_{AO_2} this can usually be readily reversed by increasing the fraction of O_2 in inspired air (F_iO_2); hence the basis of oxygen therapy.

Depending on the magnitude of surgery, this effect may be short lived for peripheral surgery (<30 minutes) but more prolonged with major upper abdominal or thoracic surgery (>3 days), especially if postoperative opioids are used (e.g. PCA).

There are a number of consequences of failing to treat low oxygen levels (Figure 34.2). However if patients' oxygen saturations are normal on air, then oxygen is not required.

Oxygen delivery devices are traditionally divided into two categories, fixed and variable performance devices.

Fixed These supply a fixed and known concentration of oxygen. The device must be able to match the patient's peak inspiratory flow rate (>30 L/min), otherwise air is entrained around the mask at times of peak inspiratory flow and resulting in an unknown inspired concentration of oxygen reaching the patient. Fixed oxygen performance devices use the entrained air from the Venturi effect (Figure 34.3) to ensure these high flow rates are delivered.

Variable These devices consist of a simple face masks and nasal prongs, which give an unknown concentration of oxygen; however, they are commonly used.

Others

Patients may need prescribing:
- anticoagulants: the timing of heparin administration to prevent pulmonary thromboembolism needs to be balanced against the risks of postoperative bleeding, especially if an epidural is *in situ*;
- antibiotics;
- insulin.

35 Anaesthesia away from the hospital setting

Sometimes anaesthesia will need to be given to patients away from the usual hospital environment. This means there will be differences in several key areas:
- isolation – an appropriate level of experience in airway management and anaesthesia is essential as back up might be a long way away, or not available at all;
- the safety of the environment – uneven ground, water hazards, roads/traffic;
- extremes of weather conditions;
- lighting;
- resources available, in terms of equipment, drugs, monitoring, power sources, assistants;
- number of staff;
- the type of patient and their injuries;
- lack or absence of investigations, e.g. X rays, lab tests;
- postoperative recovery facilities.

Examples of locations include isolated clinics, road or rail traffic accidents, and military engagements. Administration of anaesthesia in isolated sites is becoming less common.

It is essential that the same standard of monitoring, equipment and recovery facilities are available as there are in a hospital setting.

Although now less commonly used, portable vaporizers are available for use in an isolated situation. Inhalational anaesthesia can be given using a drawover vaporizer to provide anaesthesia in remote locations. It functions by using air, with or without supplemental oxygen, being drawn over a vaporizer and from there to the patient. The patient's own respiratory effort or a self-inflating bag drives the system. Desirable features include having low internal resistance to gas flow and the ability to deliver a constant concentration of volatile anaesthetic despite changes in the patient's minute volume or the operating temperature. It has the advantages of being: portable, cheap and simple design, no need for pressurized fresh gas flow and robust.

Trauma

The important factors in a trauma situation include:
- safety of rescuers;
- stabilization of patient (ABC and primary survey; see Chapter 25);
- transport;
- definitive treatment.

The 'golden hour' is a term used to emphasizes the critical importance of early treatment after injury when rapid medical intervention is most likely to save life and limit major morbidity. It is more likely that it is intervention and patient treatment as soon as possible, rather than the specific first 60 minutes, that is key.

The term 'scoop and run' is used to describe the transfer of a patient from the site of injury to the site of definitive treatment as soon as practical and, if available, to a trauma centre, as happens in the UK and USA. Some countries practise a longer physician-led assessment and treatment at the trauma scene (so-called 'stay and play') before transfer to hospital (e.g. in France and Belgium).

Emergency treatment given at the scene will include drugs to facilitate endotracheal intubation, typically ketamine and suxamethonium, as well as morphine for analgesia and vasopressor agents if indicated (e.g. adrenaline).

Surgical intervention at the incident scene might have to take place (e.g. limb amputation as part of extraction, emergency thoracotomy for penetrating chest injuries, chest drain insertion).

Intravenous access might prove difficult and the intraosseous (IO) route can be used successfully in adults with major haemorrhage as a means of fluid resuscitation and drug administration. Access sites include sternum, proximal tibia and humeral head. The IO route can be used for all drugs, fluids and blood products and can be quicker to establish in an emergency situation.

Battle scenarios

In military engagements, the types of injury seen differ both in mechanism and extent from those seen routinely in a district general hospital, and include:
- ballistic injuries from firearms;
- blast injury;
- burns;
- multiple penetrating injuries;
- biological, chemical and radiation injury.

Anaesthetists play a central role in prehospital care as part of the Medical Emergency Response Team (MERT) as well as in field hospitals. A MERT consists of a medical team (usually an anaesthetist, accident and emergency specialist and two medics) as well as soldiers acting in a protective capacity, a Quick Reaction Force. On arrival, the MERT provides resuscitation, assessment and treatment, which continues on the way back to the field hospital where definitive treatment can occur.

Key points of battle trauma include:
- different mechanism of injury;
- <C>ABC approach to resuscitation;
- ongoing unsafe environment;
- transport at high speed to site for definitive treatment, e.g. low/fast flying helicopter and/or by vehicle across uneven terrain.

<C> Indicates catastrophic haemorrhage; treatment includes the use of tourniquets to stop bleeding from a limb injury (e.g. traumatic amputation, direct pressure and haemostatic field dressings). These dressings can be impregnated with haemostatic agents such as Celox™ (Medtrade Products Ltd, Crewe, UK), which forms a pseudo-clot on contact with red blood cells and tissue fluid to help stem bleeding.

Interventions that might be performed before transport to a place of safety include intubation, chest drain insertion, thoracotomy, limb amputation and arresting major haemorrhage. Early use of blood and blood products is advocated and they are given at an earlier stage than in hospital practice. The casualty is transported to a field hospital for ongoing resuscitation and definitive treatment.

Anaesthesia at a Glance, First Edition. Julian Stone and William Fawcett.

'Mass casualties' refers to the situation when the number of injured patients overwhelms the medical resources available. In this situation, treatment decisions have to be made to achieve the biggest impact on the highest number of casualties. Casualties are triaged on a four-point priority (P) scale:

P1 those needing immediate life-saving resuscitation and/or surgery, e.g. airway obstruction, haemorrhage, amputations;

P2 those needing early resuscitation and/or surgery, but some delay is acceptable, e.g. open fractures, burns covering 15–30% of the body;

P3 those who require treatment but where a longer delay is acceptable, e.g. lacerations, simple fractures;

P4 hold – those multiple-injured casualties who are not expected to survive are given supportive treatment (e.g. analgesia) compatible with the resources available, e.g. serious head injury, spinal injury;

Deceased.

Although mass casualties are thankfully a rare occurrence, it is important that all anaesthetists are aware of their prehospital management in these situations and are also familiar with the local major incident plan that all hospitals have in place.

Index